International Council of Nurses

Nursing Leadership

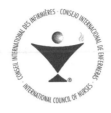

International Council of Nurses
Nursing Leadership

SALLY SHAW, MPH, BN

International Nurse Consultant
Nursing Leadership and Health Policy
Geneva, Switzerland
and Whakatane, New Zealand

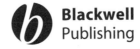
Blackwell
Publishing

Blackwell Publishing editorial offices:
Blackwell Publishing Ltd, 9600 Garsington Road, Oxford OX4 2DQ, UK
  Tel: +44 (0)1865 776868
Blackwell Publishing Inc., 350 Main Street, Malden, MA 02148–5020, USA
  Tel: +1 781 388 8250
Blackwell Publishing Asia Pty Ltd, 550 Swanston Street, Carlton, Victoria 3053, Australia
  Tel: +61 (0)3 8359 1011

First published 2007 by Blackwell Publishing Ltd

ISBN: 978-1-4051-3523-8

Library of Congress Cataloging-in-Publication Data
Shaw, Sally.
    International Council of Nurses : nursing leadership/Sally Shaw.
      p.; cm.
    Includes bibliographical references and index.
    ISBN: 978-1-4051-3523-8 (pbk. : alk. paper)
    1. Nursing services–Administration.   2. Leadership.   3. Nurse
administrators.   I. International Council of Nurses.   II. Title.
III. Title: Nursing leadership.
    [DNLM: 1. Nursing, Supervisory–organization &
administration.   2. Leadership.   3. Nurse's Role.
WY 105 S536i 2007]
RT893S528 2007
362.17–dc22

                                                2006028215

A catalogue record for this title is available from the British Library

Set in 10/12.5pt Times NRMT by Graphicraft Limited, Hong Kong
Printed and bound in Singapore by Utopia Press

For further information on Blackwell Publishing, visit our website:
www.blackwellnursing.com

Contents

Foreword

While change and chaos whirl about us, one thing agreed across borders and nations is the need for skilled leaders, adept at leading increasingly diverse teams in uncertain times and situations.

In the chaos of health care in these early years of the twenty-first century, the subject of leadership in nursing has never been more important. We are living on the edge, with increasing complex patient care, demand and costs, changing needs, competition, and an emphasis on quality. Competent, caring leaders are crucial.

This new, easy to read text, could not have come at a better time. Filled with current theory, stimulating international vignettes, and practical examples, it will be highly appreciated by new and seasoned leaders, mentors and faculty. Clearly, leadership can be learned as the author aptly illustrates through examples drawn from the Leadership for Change™ programme, by which the International Council of Nurses is helping to build a cadre of leaders for these times of constant change.

Nursing Leadership illustrates that today's leaders need to be proactive, innovative, confident, competent, strategic, flexible, and collaborative critical thinkers, who see the big picture and are prepared to mentor and be mentored. They are results-oriented individuals who lead by example and understand that leadership is about responsibility. They persevere, communicate and, most of all, they care about the issues, outcomes, goals and vision. They have their head in the clouds and their feet on the ground.

This is a book for those committed to doing better. Mixing theory with international examples, it will help readers grasp what others have experienced and accomplished. The international element is an important contribution, showing the differences of culture, politics, and societies and the similarity of our issues and our reactions.

Nursing Leadership exemplifies the attributes of its author who "walks the talk" when it comes to leadership. Both the "soul" of leadership and Leadership for Change are evident. Her passion for the topic and people, and her interest in the big picture and new experiences radiate throughout the book.

Leaders need not only to lead on the job, but also to be reflective, to have a capacity for aloneness as Stephen Covey would say. This capacity helps them see connections, ask questions, be strategic, align people and processes with the vision and mission, and to motivate others to act. These three leadership roles – path finding, aligning and empowering – are critical in today's globalised, constantly changing health care environment.[1]

Leadership development provides a positive return on investment for the individual, organisation, employees and, most of all, patients and families. *Nursing Leadership* is an important element in building such returns.

Judith A. Oulton
Chief Executive Officer
International Council of Nurses

Reference

(1) Covey, S.R. Three roles of the leader in the new paradigm. In: *The Leader of the Future* (eds Hesselbein, F., Goldsmith, M. & Beckhard, R.). Jossey-Bass, San Francisco, 1997, pp. 149–59.

Acknowledgments

This book is about leadership and leadership development, but it is illustrated with examples and case studies from the International Council of Nurses (ICN) experience with their Leadership for Change™ (LFC™) project in over 50 countries worldwide. Therefore, thanks are first due to ICN for giving me incredible experience in developing and implementing the ICN LFC™ initiative. To Connie Holleran, Executive Director who brought me to ICN, and to Judith Oulton, Chief Executive Officer, who provided leadership and support over many years, my thanks and appreciation. Subsequently, Stephanie Ferguson became the LFC™ program director, and I thank her for being a good friend and colleague, and for contributing much of the material on the LFC™ program used for examples and case studies for the period following my move from full time to part time with ICN, in 2003. Thanks also to other ICN friends and colleagues who have assisted in different ways.

The work of the LFC™ Evaluation Advisory Committee and contracted experts is greatly appreciated, and material from their various documents contributed data to this book: James Buchan (Scotland), Anne McMurray (Australia), Ligia de Salazar (Colombia), György Siminics (Geneva), Wendy Kitson-Piggott (Trinidad and Tobago), Judith Oulton (Geneva) and Jacques Gaude (Geneva).

The following people reviewed the draft manuscript and provided valuable insights and suggestions: Gay Williams, Marie Burgess and Margaret Green in New Zealand; Judith Oulton and Stephanie Ferguson in Geneva.

Appreciation and thanks are due to colleagues at Blackwell Publishing Ltd. in the UK for their assistance and support, and for arranging for valuable comment from reviewers on the initial draft book outline.

Finally, a debt of gratitude to the participants, mentors, regional team leaders, program coordinators, partners, stakeholders including national nurses' associations and governments, the World Health Organization and other funders and colleagues in the ICN LFC™, and to many others. They have contributed to the ICN LFC™ program experience from its inception in 1996 to the time of writing, and through this have added richness to the text in the examples and case studies from across the world. They have shared their leadership journeys and contributed to the book in ways too numerous to count.

Sally Shaw
Geneva, Switzerland, and Whakatane, New Zealand
2006

Introducing this book

What the book is about

This book is about effective leadership, and the development of nurses for leadership in changing and often difficult environments. This is not a book about management, but it does discuss differences between leadership and management, promoting the idea of leadership as an integral part of management in complex organizations and changing environments. The book references and uses for illustrative purposes the International Council of Nurses (ICN) experience with their Leadership for Change™ (LFC™) program[1] in over 50 countries and in a wide range of socio-political, economic, and cultural contexts. Key principles and messages are illustrated with case studies and vignettes from experience in many countries. Thus nurses tell of their own experiences – what has been important in their individual leadership journey, what has helped them, what has held them back, and what contributions they have been able to make to organizational or country developments. These experiences help reinforce the principles of effective leadership that remain constant across many different settings.

It is important to note that the selection of examples used to illustrate the text was influenced by:

- The stage of an ICN LFC™ program in a country, and the number of years it has been operating which is important when discussing outcomes and their sustainability.
- The data available, including documentation and responses to additional requests to past participants for material.
- The need for confidentiality, such as with primary data in responses to questionnaires in evaluation studies.

Wherever practical the names of the country or region are given for the examples used, to help demonstrate similarities in a cross-cultural context. However, where the examples are best not named for some reason, yet are good teaching examples, the names are not given to protect the country's anonymity.

1

Leaders on the edge

An underlying premise of this book is that nurse leaders, like others, are *leaders on the edge*. This reflects the concept of 'living on the edge'[2] which describes the leadership challenge in today's world. It means that leaders are being faced with the need for massive change because of complex events and chaotic developments throughout the world. Small 'tweaks' or incremental changes in organizations are often not enough, and sometimes only major or profound change will achieve the results needed. And in turn, more change often brings more uncertainty and anxiety. So the new realities for health care systems throughout the world are complexity, continued change, and often a certain level of chaos. Health systems have been moving toward 'the edge' as rising need and demand for health care, and rising costs, mean choices must be made as regards what health care to deliver and how to deliver it, so that countries can have effective health services that they can afford. Living on the edge means that many health care systems had (or have) two basic choices:

- Going to a higher level of complexity by changing in a profound way.

Or

- Failing to make any progress, by refusing to let go of the status quo.[3]

Many countries across the world have made the first choice. This has meant a major transformation in several of these countries, even though it has often been radical and uncertain. Leaders on the edge have had to ask what sort of health service they want for the people of their country. And if the answer has meant massive change, then leaders on the edge have had many challenges:

- accepting they cannot live with the status quo
- needing to make major changes in thinking and behavior
- learning how to manage change
- continuing to look for opportunities, even when the issues seem enormous
- being proactive, not reactive
- learning to seek solutions, not re-define problems
- being continually focused on, and responsive to the external environment
- working with and through other people, encouraging and supporting them
- accepting the responsibility of developing new leaders.

Leadership in challenging environments

For health care leaders, and many others, the complexity of the organizations and systems they work in creates a challenging environment. Recent authors have been exploring 'complexity science' as it relates to health care. This looks at the many different aspects of living [organizational] systems that are neglected or understated in traditional approaches.[4] Thus complexity science explores the unpredictable, disorderly and unstable aspects of organizations, and helps understanding of these.[5] For example, viewing leadership in health care organizations in terms of traditional command and control structures does not allow for the rapid responses and changes needed for health care improvements. The idea that organizations have to be viewed as complex adaptive structures in environments of rapid change is discussed further in later chapters.

For leadership in these kinds of organization, the development of leaders is not just about knowledge and skills, it is also about developing leadership behaviors and different ways of thinking. This may at times be painful. Leadership can be painful too, but it also has huge rewards. The leaders who make a commitment to themselves and to other future leaders have a challenging and exciting time ahead of them on their leadership development journey. They often live with continued change where they learn to find new ways of doing things, and to think creatively and strategically about how to achieve their goals.

Finding new ways of doing things has been explored in some recent research. One example looked at the relation between management practice and resident outcomes in a health care organization for elderly people. It concluded that improved and open communication and better interaction (such as staff participation in decision-making, strong relationship skills, and less command and control) are needed for better resident outcomes, explaining these results in terms of complexity science.[6]

So this book is about effective leadership, and also about what makes leadership development programs work effectively. It is about how to get good outcomes for both individuals and health services, and how to sustain these outcomes in order to realize a good return on the initial investment. The context is leadership in and for change. It applies to both organizations that respond to changing environments by changing themselves, and also to relatively stable state organizations that operate in changing environments and under economic constraints but are slower to make changes themselves.

Although much of the focus is on resource-limited health systems and settings, the book aims to demonstrate just what can be achieved in – and despite – such settings and their limitations. It also seeks to illustrate commonalities across different cultures, socio-political systems, and economic environments. Positive outcomes, results and longer-term impacts are often determined not only by the environment but also by the people in those environments – their attitudes, their skills, their confidence, their motivation and commitment. In short, their leadership skills and effectiveness. Of course one might argue that people *are* part of the environment. But the point is to demonstrate that the people who are the leaders trying to bring about improvements and change, are the people who will use their personal skills to influence and motivate others around them so they become committed to working to a common goal whatever the cultural, political, social, or economic context.

Focus and content

This book aims to be an easy-to-read informative 'text' about leadership and leadership development. It is based on experience with a wide variety of leaders and with many leadership development programs in diverse environments. It promotes the importance of balancing leadership theory and knowledge with the development of leadership attitudes, skills, and behaviors. And it explores those factors in the environment that might hinder leadership effectiveness on the one hand, or on the other hand promote positive outcomes that have real impact and are sustained in the longer term.

Globalization, health reform, ever-changing environments – all of these are big concepts, and all ultimately impact on nursing leadership. Effective leaders look beyond their immediate boundaries and work environments. They assess potential impacts on health as well as on the health sector. They are in tune with the socio-political environment and know how to both use and influence it effectively. They are aware of helping and hindering factors that influence the health sector and nursing, and develop appropriate strategies. They seek and maintain networks and partnerships in the broader environment. These ideas will be introduced in more detail in Chapter 1. Chapter 2 discusses what leadership is *not*. Chapters 3 and 4 introduce the framework of leadership used in this book, that is, the person who is the leader, the setting of leadership, and the followers. The concept of 'soul' in leadership is also introduced, and will be used in different places throughout the text.

Leadership concepts and attributes that remain constant in both rapidly changing and slower changing systems, and across different cultural contexts, will be discussed. For example, all these situations demand an understanding of the broader health and social system within which nursing functions. This knowledge is used to influence policy and management decisions which requires skills in policy development, negotiation, oral and written communication, and attributes such as confidence and the ability to inspire confidence in others. Examples will be used from different settings to illustrate similarities in approach, across countries and cultures, to the use of leadership skills and behaviors such as being strategic, negotiation skills, motivating others, and demonstrating confidence in presenting well researched proposals and options.

Change can be developed from within or imposed from without. In both situations nurses can play an important role, depending on their leadership and management skills. The premise is taken in this book that leadership and management are separate, yet interconnected concepts. In Chapter 3, the concept of effective leadership is described as having a clear vision or view of the future and future goals and having the ability to motivate others toward achievement of those shared future goals. A number of leadership attributes and components are incorporated into effective leadership, such as strategic thinking, confidence, engendering confidence and trust in others, and excellent communication and interpersonal relationships.

Similarly, in change management, the 'managers', 'executives', 'leaders' of the organization, must possess the above attributes. But in bureaucratic centralized organization where change is slow, the manager is usually more of an administrator who ensures tasks and activities are completed and the organization runs smoothly on structured lines. Between these two poles there is any number of combinations, and the manager who is right for one type of organization will not be right for another. The person who manages a changing organization in an environment of change must have leadership skills and attributes. That same person would probably be bored and frustrated managing a stable-state organization. On the other hand, a person who is excellent in a stable-state organization could find it difficult to manage in a changing dynamic organization. They may need to control everything themselves and become stressed and ultimately unable to cope. Different types of organization will therefore be discussed, including the leadership and management styles appropriate for different types of settings. Both must be understood if appropriate career decisions are to be made.

To get the most from this book, it is important to appreciate how the term leadership is used. It does not just refer to 'the top'. It is not about positional leaders. Clinical leaders, team leaders, project leaders, and others – all are leadership roles, and all need leadership skills and attributes.

While the book has been written to flow as a whole, it is also designed so the readers can focus on a particular section relevant to their needs. For example, Chapters 3 and 4 focus on the concept of leadership, while Chapters 5 and 6 focus on leadership development programs and what helps make them effective. The same framework of person, setting, and followers is used in both chapters because leadership development is not just about the person, but must take the environment (the 'setting') and the followers into account. Some programs must, in fact, actively involve them, if they are to be successful.

An essential component of leadership development programs is helping students/participants recognize the need to address those factors in their immediate and broader environments that might help or hinder their continued development as leaders. It is not enough to gain some knowledge about leadership, or complete a leadership development program, if the results and outcomes are unlikely to be sustained in the longer term. On an individual level it may be ongoing mentoring or structured planning for individual development that is required. Perhaps a new role or position will provide the opportunity to practice and sustain newly developed attitudes and skills. Perhaps assistance is needed with strategies to deal with negative environmental factors that might seem just too formidable to tackle.

Leadership in practice, and outcomes from leadership development, for the person, the setting (the environment), and the followers will be discussed in Chapters 7 and 8. Chapter 9 explores the whole question of sustainability of outcomes. In Chapter 10, leadership and leadership development are considered within the context of 'success'. It suggests ten categories to define success in leadership development of nurses:

(1) Contribution to health policy
(2) Focus on quality
(3) Impact on organizations
(4) Networks, partnerships, and strategic alliances
(5) Community development
(6) Ongoing education of self and others
(7) Curricula change
(8) Strengthening of national nurses' associations
(9) Leadership behavior and 'soul'
(10) Return on investment

Chapter 10 also asks the question: How is a good return on investment obtained in these days of financial constraints? Return on investment is considered, with case studies to illustrate, in the context of the following categories:

- High return (high/high)
- Medium return
  - high/low
  - low/high
- Low return (low/low)

Much of Chapter 10 is presented in 'list' format, to help readers review and monitor their own, or others', leadership practice more readily. Experiences from the field help emphasize the keys to success. Finally, Chapter 11 briefly reminds readers of the impact that nursing leadership can have, both individually and collectively.

At the end of each chapter there is a section on 'Exercises and discussion questions'. Readers are encouraged to select what are most relevant to them. It is further recommended that the suggestions to write down specific ideas, or to discuss things with a group, are followed, because it is in this way that critical and analytical thinking can be developed further, and the benefits of peer review considered against self-assessment.

Summary of purpose

To summarize, the purpose of this book is to provide an easy-to-read text on leadership and leadership development that is equally suitable for readers who have English as a first or a second language. The book emphasizes the relationship of leadership and leadership development programs to environment and change. It is aimed at leaders of all levels and in different politico-economic and cultural settings, and at educators responsible for leadership development programs. It seeks to demonstrate commonalities across cultures. The text is illustrated with quotes, case studies and other data drawn from experience with the ICN LFC™ program in over 50 countries.

Although written primarily for nurses, the messages are equally relevant for other professions. Thus the main target audience is nurses and others in a range of health care settings including clinical leaders, and teachers and students in a variety of leadership development programs run by consulting institutes, universities, hospitals, and others. While the focus is on the health system, it is hoped that other readers will find information in this book that will help them on their own journey to becoming strong and effective leaders . . . for the journey is significant, and it is lifelong.

The leadership development journey

'There is absolutely no doubt in my mind that involvement in this program has forced participants to be more proactive, to try new ways of operating, to be better communicators, to set new horizons, to feel empowered enough to go after the challenge rather than running from it . . .'[7] (Caribbean)

'Some participants already stand out as leaders. They accept responsibility, take initiative, are demonstrating their effectiveness, and go that extra bit further to maximize their learning and development.'[8] (United Arab Emirates)

There is an old Chinese proverb, 'The journey of a thousand miles begins with one step.' This book is about taking that step . . . beginning the journey.

References and notes

(1) Hereafter called ICN LFC™.
(2) Fitzgerald, L.A. (1994) *Living on the Edge*. The Benchmark.
(3) *Ibid.*
(4) Zimmerman, B., Lindberg, C. and Plsek, P. (2001) *Edgeware: Insights from Complexity Science For Health Care Leaders.* Texas, USA: VHA, Inc.
(5) *Ibid.*, p. 7.
(6) Anderson, R.A., Issel, L.M. and McDaniel, R.R. (2003). Nursing homes as complex adaptive systems: relationship between management practice and resident outcomes. *Nursing Research*, 52 (1), 12–21.
(7) Regional Project Leader, Report on LFC™ Project Caribbean Region, 16 January 2000. ICN, unpublished.
(8) Report to World Health Organization (WHO), ICN, and Director of Nursing, Ministry of Health, United Arab Emirates, March 2003. ICN, unpublished.

Chapter 1
Background: the challenge of change

The health environment

For some years, health services across the world have been under threat. Resources are often limited, and demand has grown. Leaders in many countries are being faced with the need for massive change. Traditional values about health care are being challenged and are often in direct conflict with the emerging 'business' environment in health, which is seen by many as the only way to cope with increasing demand and increasing costs.

A number of factors contribute to the need for change, but their weighting often varies between countries or regions. The broader issues include:[1]

- aging populations (to a greater or lesser extent in different countries) which increase both the demand for and cost of different types of health care service
- increase in the size of some health issues and problems, and emergence of new ones
- the need to determine priorities for health care spending and what is affordable
- economic constraints on what resources are available for health care
- providing quality care within these economic constraints
- public attitudes and expectations
- the effectiveness of public policy in health
- accessibility to health services through either affordability or geography
- operational, managerial and financial issues.

Operational, managerial and financial issues in health care organizations and systems are highlighted in Box 1.1.

Today's complex health environment is global. It is global in the sense that many of the major influences on health systems go beyond national boundaries. Examples are:

- Global trade and changes in markets
- Regional trade agreements
- National debts and trade deficits
- Workforce diversity and cross-boundary migration
- Information technology and communications
- International donors (of health dollars and expertise)
- Transnational health care companies.

Among the pressures on health systems are the impacts of globalization. However, globalization also provides many opportunities. Historically, the concept of globalization has been tied to trade and related economic issues and trends. It is now generally considered to be much broader including political, technological and cultural dimensions, and influenced by modern information technology and communications. The 1999 UN Human Development Report emphasizes that globalization is a growing interdependence of the world's people more than the flow of money and commodities.[2] In addition, this report highlights both the opportunities for human advance and the threats created by globalization.

The opportunities include increased trade, new technologies, foreign investments, and expanding media and internet connections. These are believed to offer enormous potential for human and economic advances and poverty eradication in the twenty-first century. Examples of new opportunities relating to the health sector, in particular arising from new technologies and expanding internet connections, are shown in Box 1.2.

The positive effects, however, are not equitably accessible to a large proportion of the world's population. Opportunities and benefits are not shared evenly. There are growing inequalities within countries, and between rich and poor countries, and new threats to human security. The negative effects, also shown in Box 1.2, are more likely to affect poorer people and countries than the richer ones.[3]

Box 1.1 Operational, managerial and financial issues contributing to health sector reform.

- Management information systems inadequate in many countries
- Strategic planning and policy development based on research and evaluation, inadequate, or absent
- Bureaucratic management systems including centralized planning and decision-making
- Lack of innovation or cost-effectiveness in health care delivery
- Service planning not integrated
- Inadequate facilities and assets with high maintenance costs
- Responsiveness to communities and stakeholders often lacking
- Inadequate development of the health workforce to meet changing needs and requirements
- Little performance measurement

> **Box 1.2 Positive and negative effects for the health sector from globalization.**
>
> | **New opportunities** | **Negative effects** |
> | --- | --- |
> | Telehealth and telenursing | Environmental pollution |
> | Increased networking and sharing of ideas and information among professionals and organizations | Faster transmission of diseases |
> | New education methodologies | Breakdown of local cultures |
> | New job opportunities | Exposure to products dangerous to health |
> | New technologies bringing improvements in health care and the quality of life for many | Spread of unsafe working conditions |

In trying to achieve a reasonable balance between the opportunities and the threats of globalization, developing countries in particular face a major challenge: how to manage their integration into the global economy, so they exploit the benefits and achieve high and sustainable growth and employment and eradication of poverty, while also minimizing the risks of economic and social dislocation, and marginalization.[4] This is the challenge of sustainable human development.

Health reform

Against this background of global linkages influencing health care and an increasingly complex health environment, many countries have accepted that incremental changes are often not enough and sometimes only major or profound change will achieve the results needed. The new realities are seen to be continued complexity and continued change. Many believe that to survive, systems must change. This is often prompted by factors both outside and within the health system.

A pressing issue has been the need to *rethink* and *restructure* the health system to try to remedy major operational, managerial, and financial problems. Health systems and organizations are challenged to find acceptable ways of defining priorities to achieve equity, quality, and efficiency. The trend in health systems of many countries is now toward regional integration or collaboration and rapidly shifting models of financing and organizing health systems.

Thus in many countries, the response to the challenges of the new environment has been health reform. These movements are usually a part of a major restructuring of business and economic systems throughout society, usually government led. In this respect health has become highly political. Health reform is a global trend, closely linked to economic policies and development. Its goal is to improve the health status of populations by getting the best value for money from available resources in the face of increased demand. It has been gathering momentum during this past decade, as the availability of funding for health care has been challenged by increased costs and increased or changing needs and demand for health care services.

A decade ago the Organization for Economic Co-operation and Development (OECD) published a review of health reform in 17 OECD countries.[5] It concluded that virtually all the 17 OECD countries faced the same problems and had common objectives concerning health care, particularly the provision of quality health care at an affordable cost. All the countries have aging populations and rising costs from new health technologies. The dynamics underlying the changes are: to increase efficiency by economic incentives and competition, often to increase consumer choice and satisfaction, and to assess quality and promote health in its widest sense.

Throughout the 1990s the work of the World Health Organization (WHO) also focused on health system reform. Reports of countries less developed than OECD countries, highlighted critical components of health system development necessary to support 'Health for All'. These include:[6,7]

- Health policy development
- Improved managerial processes
- Community involvement
- Inter-agency and inter-sector cooperation
- Tracking and monitoring health reform process and outcomes
- Creating internal markets and managing relations with the private sector
- Financing
- Decentralization
- Interactions between health and other sectors including the public sector
- Capacity building
- Policies and aid.

Strategies of health system reform vary in different countries. Most often they involve:

- changes in health policy
- 'restructuring' of health care services and organizations.

These two categories can include a wide range of activities. Examples are:

- decentralization, with greater emphasis on accountability and performance management
- changes to the system of financing health care
- privatization
- separation of service funder, purchaser and provider
- cost containment strategies such as rationing and managed care

- management improvements such as monitoring and measurement of performance and outputs, computerized systems to cost services and manage information, changes to the level and mix of staff, and a focus on better education and development for managers.

Health reform usually involves profound change. Reform impacts on both providers and consumers of health care services. Nurses have often been negatively affected by health reform, especially if the main emphasis has been on cutting costs. Often nurses have borne the brunt of this and have experienced conflicts between productivity demands, safety and quality within reduced staffing and resources. For many health professionals, health reform can be threatening or challenging. It often requires new ways of doing things. However, in many instances health reform has had positive impacts. It has resulted in more services being provided and more health needs being addressed in a number of countries. Innovations and improved quality have been observed in different situations. And in many countries undergoing fairly significant health system changes, nurse leaders are accepting the challenge of a different type of education which will equip them to become equal partners with other health care leaders and managers. Many have moved to include broader responsibilities in their nurse leader roles, while others now accept leadership responsibilities in health that may or may not include nursing.

Health systems that change more slowly

Although some countries have responded to the pressure of changing environments with health reform, in others the health systems have remained highly bureaucratic and centralized, with values and mind-sets reflecting those of the system in which people operate. This was referred to in the introduction to this book, in the context of complexity science, where it was noted that looking at leadership in health care organizations in terms of traditional command and control structures does not allow for the rapid responses and changes needed for health care improvements. In fact, to focus less on prediction and control and more on fostering relationships and conditions where complex adaptive systems can develop, makes it more likely that creative outcomes will be produced.[8] In centralized and controlling systems, nurses are often marginalized. They may perceive themselves, and be perceived by others, as relatively powerless to influence health policy, improvements and changes. This applies at all levels of the health system. In such circumstances, change is often difficult, but certainly not impossible. Leaders are emerging who seek to change systems from within the constraints of their environments.

The more minimal changes adopted by such countries can be tied up with the degree of political stability, level and type of education of leaders and managers, personal and economic power, the status of women in society, and the image of different health care provider groups such as nurses. Another key factor is often the presence of bureaucratic personnel systems that still support the acquisition of leadership roles and positions based on length of service rather than on merit and leadership ability. These situations both support and are made possible by long-standing centralized systems that those at the top are often reluctant to change. Such centralized and often bureaucratic systems may have suited stable environments in the past, before the burgeoning costs of health care and the influence of advanced technology. But they have generally proved unable to respond effectively and quickly to the pressing challenges facing health organizations today.

Implications for nursing and nurses across countries and cultures

Whether nurse leaders operate in a system of health reform, or of relatively unchanging and centralized bureaucracy, the challenges are often similar albeit different in expression. In both situations the need for effective and strong nurse leaders is clear. The more critical requirements for nurse leaders are listed below and illustrated with data from the International Council of Nurses Leadership for Change™ (ICN LFC™) program reports and other documents from different countries and cultures, reflecting the cross-cultural relevance of key issues and requirements for nursing leadership in challenging times.

The critical requirements of nurse leaders discussed below are:

- understanding of the broader health and social system within which nursing functions
- external awareness
- able to use the benefits of technology
- contributing to and influencing health and public policy
- motivating and encouraging others to positive action
- being well informed and strategic in their thinking and action
- working with others to achieve common goals
- assessing and developing new opportunities for nursing
- being proactive in implementing training and education geared to the changing world
- adapting and developing new roles and new skills as health systems change.

(1) *Nurse leaders must have an understanding of the broader health and social system within which nursing functions.* This is one of the most important attributes of a nurse leader and manager. It includes the development of skills in working effectively with the media, thus linking nursing to the broader health and social system of the country.

Understanding the broader health and social systems

'Our thoughts have definitely been redirected as far as health reforms are concerned, and what is taking place globally . . . also leadership attributes which we thought were not applicable to nursing, such as political skills . . .'[9] (East, Central and Southern Africa)

(continued overleaf)

'I have been involved in evaluation of sustainability of a program at regional level . . . this has involved creating an evaluation model with other health professionals towards promoting health, taking a perspective of implementation at national level . . . and sensitization of health professionals on the development and sustainability of management ability through leadership.'[10] (Latin America)

(2) *Nurse leaders must have good external awareness.* This is necessary to understand the interrelationship of the many complex socio-political factors that impact on health and prepare themselves for the new environment.

External awareness

'It is a challenge to adapt to and perform in a new system that encourages risk-taking, creative innovations and new development.'[11] (Samoa)

'. . . political skill, negotiation and influence were not viewed by me as essentials for leadership roles. However that view has since been changed . . . This learning will be particularly useful because of the many challenges confronting me and my colleagues in our country, including ethnic and political issues. I will certainly need to take on a more proactive leadership role.'[12] (Caribbean region)

(3) *Nurse leaders must be able to use the benefits of technology.* This includes technology in clinical systems, technology in management such as computerized financial and performance monitoring systems, and communication technology such as computers and the internet.

Using technology

In Bangladesh, Myanmar and Nepal, Vietnam, Mongolia, Yemen and in other countries, nurse leaders are recognizing the importance of learning computer technology, and communicating and networking through email and the internet. A significant proportion of objectives in participant Individual Development Plans (IDPs) in these countries result in learning activities related to this technology.[13] (Asia and Middle East regions)

'The mission (of the regional team project) . . . is to develop an information system, which will integrate existing databases in the areas of education, professional practice, legislation and research, among others. This will support effective nurse leadership in the Southern Cone region and Brazil.'[14] (Brazil/Southern Cone region)

(4) *Nurse leaders must have the ability to contribute to, and help influence, health and public policy.* This continues to be an issue for nursing. Nurse leaders consistently report their concerns about lack of involvement in health policy, or lack of skills to contribute effectively, or both. The nursing profession has the potential to be a strong political force, but needs to systematically apply itself to influencing decisions and shaping health and social services. It can influence political decisions such as the allocation of resources and priorities for spending. And because nursing provides essential services and

is knowledgeable about client needs and health care issues, it should be contributing to the planning and organizing of health care services. To do this, nursing must be alert to possible changes in policy and health care services, and be active in making representation to governments and planning committees.

More often success in influencing policy is seen at an organizational level, such as a hospital or education institution. However, nurse leaders in government, if they have the skills to do so, can significantly influence top-level government policy. To do this they must recognize the skills required in influencing public policy, and prepare themselves for this role. It becomes more difficult in systems in which senior nurses in government are still promoted on the basis of length of service, often very close to their retirement date – this makes strategic thinking and activities based on longer-term goals difficult if not almost impossible. In such systems, it may rest with other levels of nurse leaders to exert influence to bring about policy change.

The first two examples in the following box show nurse leader involvement in and influence on policy at both the macro (national) and the micro (hospital) level. The third example describes the role of the professional nursing association in preparing both nurses and the nurses' association for a greater role in health policy.

Influencing policy

'I engaged myself in an academic research study entitled "A study to determine the reasons for the non-appointment of senior nurse leaders to policy-formulation positions in the ministry . . .". The study opened up further my understanding of policy-formulation and related issues, and the policy-formulation process. I was able to use the findings to make representations to the Public Services Commission (PSC) for the recognition of nurses' contribution to health. The PSC accepted the recommendations of the study and have made some changes. Capable senior nurse leaders have been identified for further training to facilitate their appointments to head policy-formulation positions in strategic units within the Ministry.'[15] (Zimbabwe)

'In [the] initial phase [of a project to implement nursing care plans] it was so difficult . . . some of the nursing staff were not motivated. To solve this problem we had workshops, re-orientation classes and counselling. To use the plan cards on a regular basis and to use compulsorily, we had [a] meeting with stakeholders (administration) and Project Advisory Committee, to make it a policy of the hospital to use nursing care plan cards. The result was that the hospital Director and Matron agreed to make policy.'[16] (Nepal)

'Input into policy impacting on nursing and health is a critical role for nurse leaders. We are encouraging all nurses, health care providers and policy makers to become a part of this [LFC™] initiative that promotes adequate preparation of nurses to meet the challenges driven by social reform. As a result of the project the Nurses Association has been strengthened and we now have established committees to review and forward recommendations on the new health laws and acts. We have gained the respect of the Ministry of Health, and the Association is now invited to serve on several National Health Committees.'[17] (Bahamas)

(5) *Nurse leaders must be able to motivate and encourage others to take positive action.* This includes making improvements in health care settings, or taking advantage of the opportunities of health reform and globalization and helping redress the more complex issues.

Motivating others to take positive action

'As my personal mentor . . . her whole attitude has been exemplary. She has demonstrated high ethical standards of a leader. She has been very understanding, flexible, approachable and dependable. She offers her guidance in a motherly manner. Her supreme support makes one do the impossible. She exercises democratic authority that accommodates everyone despite the difficulties she faces. Her zeal to overcome challenge is an enkindling spirit to her subordinates.'[18] (Zambia)

'An evaluation in one project country confirmed that a significant number of nurses who have now received some leadership training, have moved into leadership positions . . . many now participate in national health policy and negotiation committees, have pursued further academic training or are anxious to receive further continuing education and/or have initiated the introduction of leadership and management courses for their staff in health care delivery settings. . . . In another country, project evaluation identified a high level of respect among fellow nurses for the leadership exhibited by nurses from the leadership development program, and younger nurses have taken up the challenge to implement projects, make presentations and take decisions. They are being selected for policy-making committees.'[19] (Caribbean region)

'In my numerous contacts with my mentor I learned to look for opportunities . . . and to be enthusiastic about helping others'[20] (Mauritius)

---

(6) *Nurse leaders and nursing must be well informed and strategic in their thinking and action.* This includes being strategic in working in partnership with the community, the media and with other organizations that have a role and interest in health.

Strategic thinking and action

'I have learned to think strategically . . . I have followed a strategic thinking model for planning, implementation, and evaluation of the project.'[21] (Honduras)

'Making strategic alliances . . . helps combat resistance to change.'[22] (Tanzania)

'One team project relates to establishing nursing strategic directions for Mongolia. They are developing human resource policies for all nurses in the country. They have started examining all nurses' roles and responsibilities, salaries, working conditions and job descriptions in their hospitals . . . and are working closely with the MOH on this project. They will make policy recommendations regarding reward systems that are fairer and more equitable, and consider nurse patient ratios, not necessarily to set a standard ratio for the country but rather to determine nursing workloads more equitably in the country . . . Participants developed a policy paper and memo to accompany the new job descriptions for Ministry of Health consideration. Their work . . . revealed that they are gaining the political and policy skills necessary to create strategic documents for review and consideration by key stakeholders in Mongolia.'[23] (Mongolia)

(7) *Nurse leaders must be able to work with others to achieve common goals.* Working with and through others is critical. Nurse leaders cannot bring people with them towards achieving a vision and key goals, unless they are able to work effectively with a range of different people at different levels.

Working with others to achieve results

'Project outcomes were a wonderful demonstration of what can be accomplished when many stakeholders put their heads and hearts together.'[24] (Caribbean region)

'I have managed to raise staff morale by networking with other stakeholders in the community to contribute toward improving service delivery . . . we have reduced the number of staff going on sick leave by 50 per cent . . . and have involved community volunteers to assist us in certain activities at the hospital to help reduce workload.'[25] (East, Central and Southern Africa region)

'Team members approached and organised local authority persons, Non-Governmental organisations (NGOs) and different health personnel, to participate actively in the project activity. This participation brought about a reduction in (TB treatment) defaulter rate.'[26] (Myanmar)

---

(8) *Nurse leaders must be able to assess and develop new opportunities for nursing.* This includes the public sector and in private practice, in consultancy, in health planning and management, and in developing new models of nursing care delivery.

New opportunities

'I see a bright future. I am very excited about my work as a consultant . . . I am making great contacts regionally and internationally and keeping myself updated and current . . . I continue to try and maintain my "keep fit" regimen and hopefully will continue to contribute to health care.'[27] (Caribbean region)

'We have established a proposal for different models to decrease the number of post-operative infections, decrease the number of days staying in hospital, and to decrease hospital costs.'[28] (Latin America region)

'The community home-based programme is very essential for the prevention of DHF (Dengue Haemorrhagic Fever) and to overcome the increased burden of hospital workload . . . the cooperation and coordination between health personnel and community is successful . . . and the knowledge of "Do and Don't" for DHF is increased. Therefore, on the previous year, the incidence of DHF in this area is significantly reduced and I greatly appreciate the effort of the project members.'[29] (Myanmar)

---

(9) *Nurse leaders must be proactive in implementing training and education geared to the changing world.* At the same time, nurse leaders must help develop skills and attitudes that will make individual nurses and nurses' associations strong, able to live with and manage change, and able to be effective change agents.

Training and education

'We have created an MA programme in nursing through distance learning.'[30] (Latin America region)

'The project team gets more interest and enquiry about ICN LFC™ programme . . . and we get more alert people in regular continuing nursing education programme.'[31] (Nepal)

'As president of the national nurses' organisation (NNA) I organized a "day of reflection" for the new Executive Committee. We elaborated a program for a whole year taking into account the various changes in the health sector and our commitment to meet the needs and aspirations of our members . . . this has enabled us to organize our activities in a very methodical manner and it serves as a guide to monitor and evaluate achievements. It has improved the image of the organization and has enabled us to recruit new members.'[32] (Mauritius)

(10) *Nurse leaders must be able to adapt and develop new roles and new skills as health systems change.* In many countries, nurses in top-level management in health organizations and in government have developed new policy advisory roles in order to contribute to health and health service improvements. This may mean giving up much of the operational management that has been their focus in the past, as that role often becomes redundant when organizations decentralize or restructure. For many nurses in government and health delivery organizations, this has meant the loss of previously held positional power. It has been a difficult transition for many to make, and not all have been successful. Sometimes this has contributed to visible nursing leadership (positional) being removed from the organization altogether.

Some nurses have made the transition to policy from operational management; others have not. In a number of instances, the jobs have been lost (or under threat) in the restructuring process, because people (including some nurses) have not sufficiently understood the role and contribution of nurse leaders in policy as opposed to operations. The following example will be familiar in many countries, and while the specific strategy here (strike) is not being advocated or endorsed in this book, it does highlight the importance of being proactive and preparing well-researched arguments for discussion with senior government officials.

Responding positively to change

'In our country, in 2002, health reforms were deepening. Within this new framework the Nursing Directorate was to disappear. Together with the NNA (National Nurses Association) CEO and a group of representatives from around the country, we decided to go to the Ministry of Health and if nothing was done we would go on strike. To do so, we based our arguments on the laws of the country and several agreements, and we succeeded in convincing the Minister to attend the group meeting and not to quit the Directorate.'[33] (Latin America)

However, it is not just the people at management level who must understand the implications of the health system changes and challenges outlined above.

Nursing collectively (such as through professional associations) must ask itself what is being done about the challenge of providing quality care within the imperatives of cost containment, efficiency and improving equity of access, including care for the more vulnerable and needy populations.

> Many ICN LFC™ team projects focus on the challenge of quality improvement in an environment of cost containment . . . The LFC™ programme for Phase 1 in Bangladesh developed its vision statement as 'By 2010 nursing will provide quality, customer oriented care within available resources, and through proper education effective leaders will contribute to health policy and planning for Bangladesh'. Note the emphasis on 'within available resources'. Team project outcomes contributed to this broad, long-term goal.[34] (Bangladesh)

We must also reflect on the impact of changes on the culture and value of nursing, taking account of the culture and values of different countries and societies, and ask ourselves how to assess and convey to others the value of nursing in a changing world. In many countries, concerns are expressed about the perceived credibility, value and position of nursing in society, and the effects of this in terms of confidence, self-reliance and motivation. These country situations can vary enormously, but require of their nurse leaders similar attributes such as courage, confidence, ability to motivate others, perseverance, strategic and long-term thinking, advocacy and effective communication.

All the examples given in the ten areas above are either a product of, or an indication of the need for, leadership development to create strong and effective nurse leaders for the challenging environment that is health care today.

Developing nurse leaders

At all levels, and in all settings, nurses need to develop new skills in leadership. This is as important at clinical team level as it is at top corporate level in an organization. Whether we are talking about health systems undergoing major or rapid change or about centralized bureaucratic systems where change may be slower, it is the premise of this book that the development of nurse leaders for both types of situation should be *in essence* the same – that is, there is:

- acquisition of a knowledge base (that may vary from country to country and from situation to situation)
- development or enhancement of skills, attitudes and behaviours. These include confidence, strategic thinking, effective oral and written communication skills, excellence in interpersonal relations, the ability to motivate oneself and others, building effective partnerships and alliances, and others.

In both situations the need for effective and strong nurse leaders is clear. And understanding the broader health and social system within which nursing functions is one of the most important attributes of a nurse leader and manager. These will all be explored in the chapters on leadership theory.

Today's leaders and managers have to acquire and focus on new skills. For some it means developing the strength and the will to not only face continued change and turbulence, but to also lead and manage in this kind of environment. For others it also means developing strength and will, but to lead and manage in relatively unchanging or slow changing environments that are nevertheless faced with similar external challenges and pressures. Both situations can be exhausting. Some people cannot sustain the level of energy and commitment needed for this type of management and leadership. Strategies for developing, sustaining and renewing leadership capabilities and skills are explored later in this book.

In recent years there has been a growing focus on changing the method of preparation of leaders and managers and on nurturing and developing young people and other potential leaders. One of the most critical challenges of the new millennium is to equip the current generation of nurse leaders to better face changing demands and challenges, and also to equip a new generation of potential leaders for the challenges ahead. The first group may need to make major changes in thinking and behaviour, or they may be eager to move away from the status quo and look for opportunities, even when the issues seem enormous. For both groups there will be the realization that leadership development is not just about knowledge and skills, it is also about developing leadership behaviours and ways of thinking. It is accepting that leadership in change can be painful at times because it challenges the very values we hold dear. But it can also have huge rewards.

Leaders must make a commitment to themselves and to future nurse leaders. Committed leaders usually have a challenging and exciting time ahead of them. For example, they:

- accept the challenge of ongoing complexity and major change
- understand that the combination of technology and information has generated a rate of change that moves stability to chaos and uncertainty to opportunity
- find new ways of doing things
- look for opportunities
- are proactive not reactive
- are creative and innovative rather than bound by traditional rules and regulations
- think creatively and strategically about how to achieve their goals.

Commitment[35]

'I have been nourishing my mind with one book a month.' (Panama)

'You can, if you believe you can.' (Costa Rica)

'I put my evaluation tool on my bulletin board, so as to check on my weak areas, and try to work on them on a daily basis.' (Zambia)

'Our team is determined . . .' (Bangladesh)

Nursing is facing massive change. The only thing we can be certain of is that the future is uncertain. Effective leadership development will help prepare nurses to operate at a high level of performance in the uncertain times ahead. The timing of this development is critical. Nurses can be involved in leadership development programs months or even years before they have real opportunities to use the range of skills they have acquired. Or they may enter programs some time before important health sector changes, which makes it more difficult to relate theory to practice. That is not to say that such preparation is not useful – indeed it is. These people will often become important initiators of organizational improvements and new practices.

People who have been through leadership development programs, and are able to use new knowledge and develop and practice new skills and behaviors in real and challenging change situations, are generally more likely to sustain their development and have a positive longer-term impact on their work situations. This is particularly true in relation to the timing of leadership development to a person's stage of career, or to an organization's stage of development.

Timing

'It came at exactly the right time for us . . . the health reforms came, and we were prepared.'[36] (Samoa)

'Training can motivate individuals and contribute to their capacity, but unless the working environment is conducive to change, little organizational improvement should be expected.'[37] (East, Central and Southern Africa)

Facing the challenge

Many of the issues and challenges outlined above have been identified in many countries for some time. And many of these same countries have identified a lack of preparedness of nurse leaders to meet the challenges. The proliferation of books and articles on leadership, and on leadership development programs in many countries, are an indication that the issues are not confined to nursing. It is a reflection of the complexity of our world and the rapidity of change that we are all facing.

The earlier response to the issues and challenges was to focus on management and on the development of effective managers. Then the focus changed to helping prepare *leaders*. In Chapter 3 a distinction will be made between 'management' and 'leadership', while at the same time emphasizing that the lines are blurred in many situations, especially where effective management in a change environment calls for leadership attributes at a high level.

From 1990 to 1995, the whole environment of nursing and health services was undergoing rapid change, with health reforms occurring in many parts of the world. The relevance of health sector reform to nursing was seen to be significant, as nurses are key health providers in both hospital and community settings. They plan services, allocate and manage resources, and contribute their knowledge of health and health needs to policy development and decisions. Nurses need to be part of the reform process. Those who are or will be in key leadership and management positions need to be adequately prepared for new and expanded roles. As noted above, they must have a good understanding of the context and purpose of health reform; a vision of how health and nursing services may develop in their countries; the ability to plan strategically and to manage change; and the strength and confidence to be proactive and fully involved in a challenging and often stressful change environment.

Many nursing organizations and education providers recognized this by developing new leadership programs. For ICN, part of their response was the development of the LFC™ program in 1995 to complement country-level educational programs. The first programs were implemented in 1996, and now over 50 countries are involved in LFC™. It has proved itself able to be adapted to the needs of a wide variety of countries and health systems, while retaining its basic methodology, based on action-learning, and requiring the full participation of participants. The degree of participant commitment, motivation and self-direction helps determine outcomes.

ICN methodology has many components of leadership development similar to programs developed by other organizations and in other settings. This is not surprising, given the external environment and the need for leaders with the skills to respond to challenge and change. Thus many programs run by universities, business schools, institutes, organizations and expert individuals usually have some core features in common: the development of a body of knowledge; mentorship; developing attitudes and skills through project work and 'learning by doing', and a focus on self-responsibility and individual development planning. In addition, many of the expected outcomes for the ICN LFC™ program are similar to other programs. Box 1.3, as an example, shows the generic minimum expected outcomes for the ICN LFC™ program.[38]

After an external evaluation of the ICN LFC™ program,[39] ICN in 2002 developed and began implementation of a Training of Trainers (TOT) program. Currently ICN remain involved in the implementation of new programs, training and credentialing selected program graduates to deliver new programs and monitoring activities and outcomes from both of these streams. A TOT case study is presented in Chapter 9.

As previously noted, this book should not be seen as a description and analysis of the ICN LFC™ program, but more of an exploration of leadership and leadership development in general, illustrated by the ICN LFC™ experience. From this experience, which crosses many different country and cultural boundaries and settings, some consistent results emerge that suggest there is development and enhancement of leadership competencies through application of specific teaching-learning principles and methodologies despite widely different political, economic and cultural settings.

A key part of effective leadership development programs is 'action learning', or learning by doing, in actual work and professional settings. Adaptation of program content to the actual environment is critical. In this way current and

---

Box 1.3   Generic minimum expected outcomes for the ICN LFC™ program.

- Be familiar with public sector and health reform proposals, developments, issues, and implications in their country
- Have a clear understanding of political and economic impacts on health
- Understand the requirements for effective organizations and management, and have developed skills to enhance both of these
- Have developed their leadership skills and attributes, and demonstrated the application of these through tangible results
- Be able to articulate the value of nursing to key stakeholders
- Understand how nursing can contribute to health policy development and have developed skills to make them more effective in this role
- Be strategic in their thinking, oriented to results, and proactive in developing strategies that contribute to health and service improvement
- Be more effective both as change agents and in managing change
- Have developed strategies to influence curriculum change and the preparation of other future nurse leaders
- Have become an active participant in relevant networks and a mentor system, and to be acting as a mentor to others
- Have developed, implemented and evaluated an important team project, and planned for continued sustainability of outcomes
- Can plan and deliver cost-effective, quality services within the constraints the country faces

---

future issues and challenges can be explored, and realistic strategies developed for dealing with these in both the short and the longer term. The quote in the box below sums up the possibilities in a range of effective outcomes from leadership development programs that will help the nurse leaders of today and in the future deal with, and be effective in, the challenges facing them.

Effective outcomes

'The project strategies have, in my opinion, had laudable impact, very significant at the level of participants' personal development and in several instances influencing improvements in health care systems. Over the past four years, I have seen participants blossom into leaders who go after their targets, who comfortably negotiate with senior decision-makers, who advocate strongly for proactive functioning of Nursing Associations and who have focused far more efficiently on personal development.'[40] (Caribbean)

The next chapter explores in more detail what it means to be a leader in today's health care environment.

Exercises and discussion questions

(1) Review the factors contributing to the need for change in health systems outlined on page 8 and in Box 1.1. Which are applicable to your health

system or to the organization you work for? If there are more than one, rank them in priority order. Find out what plans or policies address the most important of these in your health organization or country.

(2) Under the heading 'Implications for nursing and nurses across countries and cultures', ten critical requirements for nurse leaders are identified. Convene a small group of nurse colleagues, and discuss these implications for nursing in your organization or country health system. Which are the most important? What strategies would you suggest for helping to address them?

(3) Make a list of the various opportunities for leadership development that are available to you. Identify and justify which ones you consider to be the most appropriate and relevant to your needs.

References and notes

(1) For much of this discussion on health reform and globalization, refer to International Council of Nurses (ICN) (2004) (developed by Sally Shaw), *Globalisation and Health System Reform: Implications and Strategies for Nursing*. Geneva: ICN.

(2) United Nations (1999) 'Globalisation with a human face.' Overview in *Human Development Report*.

(3) Lister, G. (2000) *Global Health and Development: The Impact of Globalization on the Health of Poor People*. UK: The College of Health.

(4) UNCTAD/UNDP (1999) *Partnership on Globalization, Liberalization and Sustainable Development*.

(5) OECD (1994) The reform of health care systems. *Health Policy Studies*.

(6) WHO (1993) *Implementation of the Global Strategy for Health Reform by the Year 2000: Second Evaluation*. Geneva: WHO.

(7) WHO (1993) Health sector reform. *Report on a Consultation* 9–10 December, and (1994) *Report on the Second Consultation* 28–29 April. Geneva: WHO.

(8) Burns, J.P. (2001) Complexity science and leadership in health care. *Journal of Nursing Administration*, 31 (10), 474–482.

(9) Participant letter (1999) to ICN on ICN LFC™ East, Central and Southern Africa. ICN, unpublished.

(10) Participant comment (2004) in ICN LFC™ longitudinal study. ICN, unpublished evaluation data.

(11) ICN LFC™ team comment (1999) after implementing a project in a new environment that emerged from a bureaucratic health system during health system reform in Samoa. ICN, unpublished.

(12) Participant report (2001) during ICN LFC™. ICN, unpublished.

(13) ICN LFC™ documentation. ICN, unpublished.

(14) Regional Project Leader's final report (2001) by the Regional Project Leader of the Brazil/Southern Cone Regional Team Project for ICN LFC™ Caribbean and Latin America Phase 2. ICN, unpublished. (This regional project initially involved four countries. One later withdrew.)

(15) Participant report (1999) to ICN on progress with ICN LFC™ Individual Development Plan. ICN, unpublished.

(16) Team project report (2005) from ICN LFC™ Nepal. ICN, unpublished.

(17) ICN LFC™ participant from the Commonwealth of the Bahamas in *Nursing in the Caribbean, a Story of Leadership* (2002) Publication prepared by Wendy Kitson-Piggott, ICN Regional Project Leader for the Caribbean team. ICN LFC™ publication.

(18) Participant report (1999) on mentorship in ICN LFC™. ICN, unpublished.

(19) Regional Project Leader's final report (2001) of the ICN LFC™ Phase 2 for the Caribbean region. ICN, unpublished.

(20) Participant report (1999) on progress with ICN LFC™ activities, Mauritius. ICN, unpublished.

(21) Participant letter (1999) to ICN LFC™ Consultant. ICN, unpublished.

(22) Country report (1999) ECSACON/ICN LFC™. ICN, unpublished.

(23) Report (2005) after the third workshop in the ICN LFC™ program in Mongolia, 2005. ICN, unpublished.

(24) Regional Project Leader (2002) Caribbean ICN LFC™. Letter to ICN. ICN, unpublished.

(25) Participant comment (2004) in ICN LFC™ longitudinal study. Geneva: ICN, unpublished evaluation data.

(26) Report (2005) on team project presentations, Myanmar. Unpublished.

(27) Participant comment (2004) in ICN LFC™ longitudinal evaluation study. Geneva: ICN, unpublished evaluation data.

(28) *Ibid.*

(29) Township Medical Officer (2005) in report of a team project for ICN LFC™ TOT Myanmar. ICN, unpublished.

(30) Participant comment (2004) in ICN LFC™ longitudinal evaluation study. Geneva: ICN, unpublished evaluation data.

(31) Team project report (2005) ICN LFC™ program in Nepal. ICN, unpublished.

(32) Participant report (1999) on progress with ICN LFC™ activities in Mauritius. ICN, unpublished.

(33) Participant comment (2004) in ICN LFC™ longitudinal evaluation study. Geneva: ICN, unpublished evaluation data.

(34) Program documents (2002) for ICN LFC™ Bangladesh. ICN, unpublished.

(35) The examples on commitment are taken from various participant reports (1998–2001) on progress during ICN LFC™ programs. ICN, unpublished.

(36) Chief Nurse Ministry of Health Samoa, comment on ICN LFC™ in Samoa.

(37) East, Central and Southern Africa College of Nursing (ECSACON) (2003) *Report on Evaluation of the ECSA Leadership and Management Programme*. Arusha: ECSACON and the Commonwealth Regional Health Community Secretariat, pp. 60–61.

(38) ICN LFC™ program documentation (1996–2005).

(39) ICN (2002) (developed by James Buchan). *Impact and Sustainability of the Leadership for Change Project 1996–2000*. Geneva: ICN. This report is based on three evaluation components: questionnaires, undertaken by Jacques Gaude (Consultant, Geneva Switzerland); documents analysis, undertaken by Anne McMurray (Consultant, Brisbane Australia); and country case studies undertaken by Anne McMurray, Ligia de Salazar (Consultant, Santiago de Cali Colombia), Wendy Kitson-Piggott (Consultant, Trinidad and Tobago) and James Buchan (Consultant, Edinburgh, Scotland). The country case studies were coordinated into a report by Jacques Gaude.

(40) Regional Project Leader comment in *Nursing in the Caribbean, a Story of Leadership*. Publication prepared by Wendy Kitson-Piggott, ICN LFC™ Regional Project Leader for the Caribbean team, 2002.

Chapter 2
What leadership is not

Before focusing on what leadership *is*, this short chapter will discuss what leadership *is not*, using the headings listed above.

Leadership is not about position

The term 'dispersed leadership' has been described as the leadership of the future.[1] This holds that there is not *a* leader, not *the* leader, but that there are *many* leaders dispersing the responsibilities of leadership across the organization. Gone are up/down, top/bottom, superior/subordinate relationships. We must be developing leaders at every level.

So leadership is certainly not about only the positions at the top of an organization. Indeed, holding a position of high status does not necessarily make one a leader. We have often seen and condemned certain behaviors in people who are in positions of authority, such as not sharing knowledge and information, not inviting ideas from others and not developing other leaders in order to protect their own position. And yet these same people who condemn such behaviors sometimes start exhibiting exactly the same themselves once they move up into higher status positions or roles. They are not leaders. They may hold positional power and authority, but this does not make them a leader.

Position and status should be less important than the actual leadership itself. We do not always see this, especially in countries and health systems where leadership positions are based entirely or primarily on length of service rather than on merit. The following example recognizes that leadership is not just about position and there are times to step aside, times where a change in the leadership is needed.

Stepping aside for others

'LFC™ participants helped the previous CNO (Chief Nursing Officer) to create a vision and plan to strengthen nurses and midwives in the country . . . she (the previous CNO) said she resigned on purpose from being Chief Nursing Officer because she believed in leadership succession planning, and she wanted others to have the opportunity to serve, to bring new blood and new ideas . . . and as the policies were now set and the strategic plan developed they were still on top. She moved aside from the position into another leadership role in the country and will be very active, with the new CNO, in supporting and coordinating the expanded TOT (Training of Trainers) initiative 2006–2009.'[2] (Tanzania)

Drucker believes that the leader is painfully aware he/she is not in control of the universe – but *is* the one ultimately responsible. He believes that leadership is not rank or privilege, but responsibility. Effective leaders are not afraid of strength in associates and subordinates, but encourage it.[3]

Having charisma does not necessarily make one a leader

. . . and it does not guarantee leadership effectiveness.[4] Drucker adds that charisma can in fact be the undoing of some leaders as it can make them inflexible, convinced of their own infallibility, and unable to change. Although effective leadership does not depend on charisma, charisma can be used positively to motivate people toward a goal or vision shared by both leader and followers. Bethel says that 'some people's missions have transformed them into charismatic leaders because of the depth and passion of their desire to make a difference'.[5] But she does say that the mission – or working toward a vision – does not depend on brilliant speaking skills or personal magnetism.[6] We also know that charisma can be used inappropriately to manipulate people into doing what the 'leader' wants, such as some cult leaders and some political leaders.

Leadership is not management (though this is qualified)

There is much in the literature about the difference between leadership and management. They are different, despite the terms sometimes being used inter-changeably. However, successful organizations faced with the need to change in complex and often chaotic environments need to integrate strong elements of leadership into the management style and organizational culture that is developed, if the organization is to be truly effective. Many writers believe that ideal corporate management implicitly incorporates both leadership and management. That is the premise followed in this book. That said, it is important to look at the main distinctions between leadership and management so we can more clearly articulate them.

Management is a process that focuses on maintaining systems to produce goods and services efficiently. It expects predictability in future development. Leadership on the other hand is seen to be prospective, defining what the future should look like and aligning the organization with a common vision, providing inspiration to achieve transformational goals.[7] This introduces the elements of forward looking, strategic thinking and a strong human factor into the idea of leadership.

Most health organizations are complex organizations. However, before the global health reform movement and the changing environment and pressures contributing to this, most health organizations were relatively unchanging and stable. They were 'managed'. This view of the management function tended to be a series of clear and connected steps:

- Planning
- Organizing
- Staffing
- Directing
- Controlling

This view of management, as an orderly set of processes suited to orderly organizations, supported Kotter's view of management as a process focusing on systems to produce goods and services efficiently. Those management components (planning, organizing, etc.) of course still exist. But today's complex organizations rarely allow and support such orderly processes without considerable problems. There may be little innovation when innovation is needed. Staff may be apathetic because they and their ideas and skills are not valued. Change may be slow when it needs to be rapid. There is lack of responsiveness to urgent needs and environmental influences. Ongoing staff development may be minimal. The reader may at this stage like to refer back to the introduction and Chapter 1, to the outline of complexity science in understanding organizational behaviour. In addition, there is a growing literature to refer to in this emerging field of study.

Modern management of complex organizations in changing environments demands much more than the traditional view of management outlined above. (Some prefer to use the term 'administration' instead of 'management' to refer to the orderly process more common to bureaucratic organizations.) Management in complex organizations is more 'alive' and involves leaders and followers at many levels and in different health care delivery situations. It requires a mixture of skills, attitudes and behaviors that are fluid in their emphasis in different kinds of settings. It is a human talent, and a collection of human skills and behaviours as shown in Box 2.1.

This type of management clearly incorporates leadership – defining what the future might be, aligning the organization with a common vision, and providing inspiration to achieve transformational goals. Key differences between leadership and management[8] are outlined in Box 2.2.

In addition to those comparisons listed, Grossman and Valiga quote Bennis and Nanus[9] as saying that management does things right but leadership does

---

Box 2.1   Management in complex organizations incorporates leadership qualities, and requires human skills and behaviors.

- How do we motivate people?
- How do we create in others a sense of trust in managers and leaders?
- How do we help and support people to be accountable?
- How do we create effective teams in which people are willing to try new ways of doing things?
- How do we network and build partnerships?
- How do we communicate effectively?

Box 2.2   Differences between management and leadership (from Grossman and Valiga[8]).

Leader/leadership	Manager/management
Allowed or selected by a group of followers	Appointed within an organizational hierarchy
Power base comes from knowledge, credibility and the ability to motivate followers	Power base is from their position of authority
Goals and vision arise from personal interests and passion	Goals and vision are prescribed by the organization
Innovative ideas are developed, tested and encouraged among all members of the group	Innovation is not necessarily encouraged, especially if it might interfere with task accomplishment
Can involve high risk	Involves low risk and maintenance of the status quo
Relative disorder seems to be generated	Rationality and control prevail
Activities are related to vision and judgment	Activities relate to cost-effectiveness and efficiency
Focus is on people, and has a long range perspective oriented to the future	Focus is on systems and structure and tends to have a short range perspective
Freedom *is not* limited to an organizational position of authority	Freedom *is* limited to an organizational position of authority

---

the right thing. A differentiation such as used by Grossman and Valiga is useful, as it helps to clarify how the same function can differ between leadership on the one hand and management on the other. However, such a differentiation is not clearcut (as Grossman and Valiga[10] acknowledge). Management does not only exist in organizations of the relatively unchanging, efficient, status quo model.

In reality, large complex organizations in changing and often chaotic environments are also managed, by managers, but with a strong component of leadership incorporated. Similarly, a hospital clinical team leader may have some management functions incorporated in their role, such as working and leading their team within a vision and goals prescribed by the organization.

What is important is to understand the basic differences and be able to define the terms you are using and what they involve. For example, as noted above, some like to use the term 'administration' rather than 'management' when referring to the role described by Grossman and Valiga above. They then use 'management' in a broader sense to incorporate leadership functions where this is a more descriptive and appropriate term. This is useful as it suggests a range of different types of organizations, from a pure bureaucratic model at one end to a complex, changing, purposeful and people-driven model at the other. The further one moves toward this latter model, the more the management reflects leadership. A nice term to describe this is what Cammock calls *managerial leadership*.[11] He believes that effective managers practice both leadership and management, often simultaneously. Both roles are important and are mutually reinforcing – but today it is leadership, not management, that is in the shortest supply.[12] This is supported by research by John Kotter (*A Force for Change*, 1990) quoted by Cammock, which concludes that many corporations are 'over-managed' and 'under-led'.[13]

Leaders in complex organizations often have a difficult challenge in getting the balance right between the management and leadership functions, particularly in relation to longer-term strategic direction. They must adapt their leadership approach to specific strategic situations rather than having a single approach. Thus the focus and strategies needed in specific settings or situations will help determine what the leadership 'looks like'.

Do not get caught in the trap of labels – understand what you mean and mean what you say. Grossman and Valiga's description will help you understand differences between management and leadership, but at the same time we must understand that nothing is so clearcut in our complex and challenging world of health care. Management and leadership are often integrated into the same role, and the extent of each may be determined by differences in the organization or the socio-cultural-political setting. What is important is to understand the distinction in terminology between administration and management, and between management and leadership. The terms must be clear to their users and appropriate to their context. This book takes the view that because most organizations still tend to describe positions in terms of management functions, such as 'General Manager', 'Managing Director', 'Chief Executive', it is useful to distinguish between administration and management so long as the term management is used when it is also meant to convey leadership requirements and attributes. In the same way, leadership roles (as opposed to positions) often have different titles. It is the expression of those roles in action that will reflect whether the incumbents are true leaders.

Leadership is not something mystical that cannot be learned

Are leaders born or made? The research of Posner and Kouzes[14] has shown that leadership is an observable, learnable set of practices. This is also an underlying assumption to this book, and the basis for the many action-learning leadership development programs that have appeared in a number of countries in more recent years. Action-learning leadership development is enlarged on in Chapters 5 and 6, where a framework developed by Posner and Kouzes is used to link live examples across many cultures and settings to the theory and practice of leadership development. Attributes and behaviors can be developed, and new skills and behaviors can also be developed. Leaders can be made – they are not necessarily born that way.

Having said that leadership can be learned, it is useful to contemplate a view that suggests that we also need to get more 'soul' into leadership. Cammock describes 'soul' as the emotion, identity and character of the leader that become important as they involve themselves in the leadership process.[15]

Soul in leadership

'It aroused in us a powerful motivation. . . .'[16] (Latin America)

'I am very excited. . . .'[17] (Caribbean)

'Her zeal to overcome challenge is an enkindling spirit. . . .'[18] (East, Central and Southern Africa)

'She has zeal and fortitude to keep LFC™ [Leadership for Change™] going despite many "political" battles in nursing and a poor economy in the country.'[19] (Latin America)

'The most brilliant vision with the clearest measurable goals will be somewhat sterile if it does not invoke a deeper sense of soul.'[20] This concept will be explored in more detail later.

Exercises and discussion questions

(1) Do you agree with the assertion in this chapter, that 'leadership can be learned, or developed'? Make a list of arguments for and against this statement.

(2) Think about 'positional' nursing leaders you have known. Write down their observable achievements. Now think about the factors that have been of less value in their leadership, and write down what you think have been the negative implications of these factors for nursing.

(3) With a group of colleagues, identify charismatic leaders you have known or read about in you country. What were their major achievements, and what factors contributed to their success?

(4) With the same group of colleagues, identify other leaders you have known, but would not describe as charismatic. What have been their achievements? What contributed to these achievements?

(5) Identify the main similarities and difference between the two groups. Keep this list handy when you read through the next two chapters.

References and notes

(1) Hesselbein, F. (2004) *Leadership Imperatives in an Age of Change and Discontinuity.* Paper presented at the New Zealand Institute of Management Conference, October, pp. 2–3.

(2) International Council of Nurses (ICN) Report (2005) from monitoring visit for ICN LFC™ TOT Tanzania. ICN, unpublished.

(3) Drucker, P. (1992) *Managing for the Future: The 1990s and Beyond.* New York: Truman Talley Books, p. 121.

(4) *Ibid.*, p. 120.

(5) Bethel, S.M. (1990) *Making a Difference: 12 Qualities that Make You a Leader.* New York: Berkley Books, p. 38.

(6) *Ibid.*, p. 38.

(7) Kotter, J. In: Ahn, M.J., Adamson, J.S. and Dornbusch, D. (2004) From leaders to leadership: managing change. *Journal of Leadership and Organizational Studies*, 10 (4), 114.

(8) Grossman, S.C. and Valiga, T.M. (2000) *The New Leadership Challenge: Creating the Future of Nursing.* Philadelphia: F.A. Davis Company, p. 10.

(9) Bennis, W. and Nanus, B. (1997) *Leaders: The Strategies for Taking Charge.* New York: Harper Collins, p. 20.

(10) Grossman, S.C. and Valiga, T.M. (2005) *The New Leadership Challenge: Creating the Future of Nursing*, 2nd edition. Philadelphia: F.A. Davis Company, p. 7.

(11) Cammock, P. (2003) *The Dance of Leadership: The Call for Soul in 21st Century Leadership.* Auckland: Prentice Hall Pearson Education in New Zealand Ltd., p. 27.

(12) *Ibid.*, pp. 6–7.

(13) *Ibid.*, p. 27.

(14) Posner, B.Z. and Kouzes, J.M. (1996) Ten lessons for leaders and leadership developers. *Journal of Leadership Studies* 3 (3), 3.

(15) Cammock, P. (2003) *The Dance of Leadership: The Call for Soul in 21st Century Leadership.* Auckland: Prentice Hall Pearson Education in New Zealand Ltd., p. 28.

(16) Participant report in ICN LFC™ program Latin America. ICN, unpublished.

(17) Participant comment (2004) in ICN LFC™ longitudinal study. Geneva: ICN, unpublished evaluation data.

(18) Participant report in ECSACON/ICN LFC™ program. ICN, unpublished.

(19) Consultant report (2005) to the author on ICN LFC™ monitoring visit in Latin America. ICN, unpublished.

(20) Cammock, P. (2003) *The Dance of Leadership: The Call for Soul in 21st Century Leadership.* Auckland: Prentice Hall Pearson Education in New Zealand Ltd., p. 28.

Chapter 3
About leadership: the person who is a leader

Much has been written about the concept of leadership. This chapter does not attempt a literature review – that would almost be a book in itself! Rather, an attempt is made to tease out some of the themes, approaches and ideas that are defining leadership thinking in our complex and often chaotic world today.

What leadership *is not* was discussed in Chapter 2. What leadership *is* is discussed in this and the following chapter using a framework of leadership as follows:

- The person who is the leader (Chapter 3)
- The setting (environment) of leadership (Chapter 4)
- The followers (Chapter 4).

This three-way focus on leadership is used throughout the rest of the book.

What leadership *is*

A 'definition' involving leader, setting and followers

If leadership is not dependent on rank or higher status positions, or on charisma, and if it is different from management and is something that can be learned, or developed, then what is it?

Norton and Smythe[1] state that 'seeking prescriptive formulas is like trying to pick up mercury with your fingers. As soon as you think you've got it, you've lost it. Leadership is not about one thing. It does not start with "this" and finish with "that". . . Definitions can be confining and restricting . . .' These authors emphasize the experience of leadership, and that the only way one can know the experience of leadership is by living it.

This book supports Norton and Smythe's view. Leadership is not defined as such, but key elements of leadership are outlined. A framework is used of the person who is the leader, the setting (environment) and the followers, to place it in a broader context. All parts of this framework must be integrated if leadership is to be successful. In addition, the experiences of real people 'living leadership' are used to bring it to life. These people are for the most part those involved in some way with the International Council of Nurses Leadership for Change™ (ICN LFC™) programs, which are based on action learning. Participants develop as leaders by living the experience, by internalizing the highs and lows of emotion that come with this experience, and by developing the skills, attitudes and behaviors that will make them more effective.

Leadership has been defined by others, probably hundreds of times. Certain themes or elements of leadership do recur: vision, communication skills, responsiveness to and initiation of change, motivating and influencing people toward shared goals, building partnerships and developing and renewing followers. So a simple way of *describing* leadership (but not *defining* it, with a beginning and an end) is that it is having vision, or a clear view of what future state to aim for, and then being able to inspire confidence and motivate others so they share the vision and goals, and will work together to try to accomplish them. Leadership is about passion and commitment and a strong belief in self and the vision or 'cause'. It is hard work. It might mean risk and sacrifice. But it can be immensely rewarding.

However, leadership does not exist in a vacuum. The idea – prevalent in the literature – is promoted in this book, that effective leadership depends partly on the person who is the leader, partly on the situation or setting and partly on the followers. This three-fold focus will be explored and illustrated in different ways, and is the framework used in later chapters, especially those on sustainability of outcomes and defining success. It is illustrated in Figure 3.1. Note the overlapping of the different circles in the figure.

This chapter explores only one aspect of this three-fold focus: the person who is the leader, although reference will be made as applicable to setting and followers. These two components will be discussed in more detail in Chapter 4.

The person who is the leader

Leadership theories

The elements of leadership that keep recurring in the literature, often in different themes or wrapped up in different 'packages', all suggest key leadership behaviors. In particular the themes shown in Box 3.1 recur.

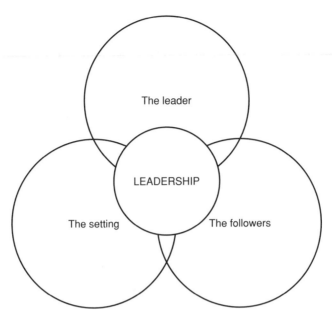

Figure 3.1   Diagrammatic illustration of leadership involving the person who is the leader, the setting and the followers.

Box 3.1   Some key leadership behavior themes that keep recurring in the literature.

- Ability to envision
- Ability to be strategic
- Confidence in self and the ability to inspire confidence in others
- Credibility and trust
- Communication skills
- Ability to motivate, inspire, influence
- Ability to take environmental, or situational, factors into account
- Ability to foster teamwork, collaboration and partnerships
- Ability to continually challenge and develop self, and foster the development of others

---

These behaviors are essential to effective leadership, but leadership is more than a list of traits or attributes. Some of the above behaviors will be more important in some settings than in others, and leaders must be able to adapt their style and strategies to suit different situations.

'Traits-based' theories are considered too limiting to give a clear and balanced picture of leadership. Indeed, more recent literature warns against leadership models that are primarily trait based, i.e. models that list a universal set of a leader's ideal qualities, personal traits or behaviors. These models need to be turned into a more dynamic model that integrates *leader*, *setting* (or situation, or environment) and *followers*. In particular 'traits theory' fails to acknowledge the importance of the situation in which leadership occurs. Ahn *et al.* say traits-based models can create resistance to change and organizational myopia. For example, they can focus leadership only on the leader at the top, such as the 'heroic leader' who is the central actor in a company's success, where leaders appear as super-men or superwomen. They consider it a paradox that while the relative value of the once celebrated individual leader is being questioned, effective corporate leadership has never been more urgently in demand or more difficult to achieve.[2]

'Situational' theory attempts to deal with the key problem of traits-based models not taking sufficient account of the *setting* of leadership. It highlights the importance of the environment and the position held, and holds that the leader is the individual who is in a position to initiate change when change is needed. However, it does not sufficiently take account of the followers.

'Transformational leadership' theory goes further by acknowledging the significant role of *followers* in the concept and practice of leadership. This approach holds that one or more persons engage with others in such a way that leaders and followers continually motivate each other to operate at higher levels. Kouzes and Posner did research in this area and came up with five types of key leadership behavior:[3]

- challenging the process (searching for opportunities, experimenting, taking sensible risks)
- inspiring a shared vision
- enabling others to act (fostering collaboration)
- modeling the way (modeling the way by their own behaviors, and setting shorter goals so the longer-term achievement seems more realistic)
- encouraging the heart (celebrating achievements and recognizing followers' contributions).

Grossman and Valiga[4] identify five recurring elements of leadership from the literature:

- Vision
- Communication skills
- Change
- Stewardship
- Developing and renewing followers

The concept of followers is a key part of transformational leadership theory.

Key leadership elements

A number of the key elements that not only relate to the person who is the leader, but also take account of the setting and the followers, will now be discussed. The elements are:

- Vision and strategic thinking
- External awareness
- Influence

- Motivation
- Confidence
- Trust
- Political skill
- Review, change and renewal of self and others
- Teamwork, partnerships and alliances

Note this is not an exclusive list, but more a description of some of the *key* elements. This should enhance a broader understanding of what it means to be a person who is a leader. As previously, examples drawn from experience with the ICN LFC™ program are given to highlight the relevance of the key elements in a variety of different countries and cultures.

Vision and strategic thinking

Many would consider that 'vision' is the most important characteristic, regardless of the setting or the leadership style required. Indeed, Drucker[5] states that the effective leader knows that the ultimate task of leadership is to create human energies and human vision. Vision can be a dream that lifts people above their routine everyday world. It introduces the passion into leadership. It means having a clear view of the future and potential opportunities. It is being able to create this clear view of the future out of major change, or from previous rigid conformity to the *status quo*. In today's environment of continual change, it is clear that organizations must not only be able to change in response to changing needs and environmental influences, but also be able to look ahead, anticipate change and plan for it. If the leaders in an organization have a clear vision of the direction it is heading in, the organization can keep focused and not be side-tracked by what may be short-term issues that may not have major long-term significance.

Vision means having long-term thinking and not being limited by the immediacy of current situations and events. Many of the great charismatic leaders of history had a very clear view of what they were working toward and an ability to keep themselves firmly focused on that long-term goal – even for years at a time. When we think of people such as Nelson Mandela and his passion for equality and social justice, Florence Nightingale and her passion to raise nursing to a skilled and respected profession, and Martin Luther King and his passion for freedom and equality of all people in his country ('I have a dream . . .'), we clearly see the vision that drove them and others who worked toward the same cause.

A vision is long term. It helps us determine the main goals to strive for along the way, and to set the short steps that will focus people on achieving the goals. So the goals are usually shorter term and allow clear plans to be made and achievable targets set. This helps keep people on track and also enables them to see how their activities fit into the broader picture. Thus the leader with vision is able to think strategically, to see the potential opportunities ahead and map out a way of getting there.

The vision should influence the entire 'constituency', such as staff of an organization, members of an association, followers of a political or philosophical movement, etc. Kouzes and Posner[6] reinforce this with their belief that leaders inspire a shared vision, meaning that they passionately believe they and other leaders (for example in the organization, or network or system) can make a difference. The leaders create an image of the future and 'give life to visions',[7] helping others to see future possibilities. This touches on the concepts of influence and motivation, which are discussed further below.

Having a vision means the leader can think long term and look beyond today and today's task and beyond the next few months . . . even beyond the horizon. It means looking at how other factors in the environment might influence the organization and its future, such as economic development, political trends, social factors, trends in health and disease, labour market trends, etc. Without a vision for the future, strategic thinking and planning is impossible and organizations get caught up in day-to-day activities that usually are not focused on longer-term outcomes. A 'goals-driven' organization based on a vision for the future is clearly distinguishable from a stable, bureaucratic organization whose goals are mainly based on providing the service or delivering the product in much the same way that they always have. The same applies for nursing. A vision for nursing means knowing what you would like nursing in your organization, or association, or country, to look like, in five or perhaps ten years time. All major programs, special projects and activities are then planned strategically to help move nursing along the path toward achieving this vision. Effective nursing leadership is the key to getting there. As Hesselbein says, it is the quality and character of the leader that determines the performance and results.[8]

Vision statements can be written in long or short versions. Longer vision statements are useful, for example, to inspire an organization or movement into a new direction. Shorter statements are often more useful for management purposes or for project planning. They can help give a clear focus to strategic (longer-term) goals focused on the vision and help focus the shorter-term action (operational) plans based on these goals. Both long and short vision statements should be inspirational, so they motivate others to working toward that vision. This provides the direction and is the driving force for effective leadership.

Vision and strategic thinking

A Tanzanian LFC™ team developed a vision that 'In five years' time there will be written Nursing/Midwifery Policy Guidelines in use by all professional nurses at all levels of health delivery, that will enhance the provision of cost-effective care for the Tanzania community'.[9] The team worked with others toward the vision and within five years the policy guidelines were in place. Subsequently Tanzania was invited to help develop standards for the World Health Organization (WHO) AFRO region, thus helping facilitate a broader regional development.[10] (Tanzania)

(continued)

'I was able to better understand the Ministry of Health's ten-year strategic planning document, and to come up with a three-year rolling plan from the document for nursing, then develop yearly and quarterly plans.'[11] (Zimbabwe)

'Having a clear vision for the future provides focus for all nursing development projects.'[12] (Latin America)

External awareness

As noted above, a leader with vision needs to be able to look at how other factors in the environment (or setting) might influence the vision and the journey toward this. This is no easy task in today's often chaotic environment – an environment of uncertainty, unpredictability and constant change. Leadership needs to take into account political and economic factors, demographic changes, new policies or new laws, health trends and issues, educational levels and other factors. This is quite a challenge, but there are a number of tools for developing both awareness and information about the external environment. Some examples are:

- 'Futures think tanks'
- Environmental scanning
- Environmental assessment
- SWOT (*s*trengths, *w*eaknesses, *o*pportunities and *t*hreats) analysis
- Assessment of helps and hindrances
- Stakeholder analysis

Following is a brief description of some of these.

Environmental scanning is a process by which an organization (or movement, or project) regularly reviews the key trends and issues that might in some way influence or impact on the organization's key activities. This can be done in meetings, workshops, by electronic canvassing of a larger audience, or by some method such as a modified Delphi technique which seeks to gather informed opinion and use this to identify key issues or set key goals or priorities.

SWOT analysis is an analysis of strengths, weakness, opportunities and threats. It helps us review the current situation and try to sort out what the future might hold. Strategies to help achieve a vision – whether they are short-term or long-term strategies – are often more effective when a SWOT analysis has been used, as specific strategies can then be developed to minimize threats or create more opportunities. Strengths and weaknesses relate to the current situation. Opportunities and threats relate to the future. It is important to appreciate that weaknesses and threats can be constraints unless they are faced and dealt with. An extremely high proportion of constraints are more perceived than real, in that they can be changed by discussion, negotiation, influence and other appropriate leadership behaviors. This requires the leader to have a positive attitude and belief that there are many things – often difficult – that can be changed by applying strategic thinking skills to find ways of overcoming, or minimizing, them. In this way, weaknesses and threats can often be turned into strengths and opportunities.

Helps and hindrances analysis is an analysis of the key factors that could influence the achievement of key goals. Specifically it assesses the positive, driving forces that will help achieve each goal and the negative, inhibiting forces that may hinder it. This gives a 'snap-shot' or picture of the current situation. As with the SWOT analysis, strategies are developed to facilitate the 'helps' and to minimize or remove the 'hindrances'.

Stakeholder analysis. Stakeholders are the individuals, groups or organizations who have an impact on, or are impacted by, what the leader or leadership sets out to accomplish. Thus a *stakeholder analysis* identifies who they are, what their interest (or 'stake') is and what assumptions can be held about them. It identifies who might be enlisted to help 'the cause' (help work toward the vision), and it also identifies those people, groups, or organizations that the leader or organization needs to work with to help them become an ally, rather than people who might block or hinder the achievement of certain goals. Examples of strategies that might be developed after a good stakeholder analysis are the formation of strategic alliances, or the assignment of specific people to manage some key relationships.

All these tools help provide different data, facts, trends, ideas and opinions, on what the future might look like and what the key environmental factors and driving forces might be that will influence this. The environmental factors might cover a very broad range – economic development, political trends, social factors, trends in health and disease, labour market trends, new developments in information technology and new ideologies.

The leader with external awareness thus has a good knowledge of how external factors might affect the organization and its future; is informed on relevant laws, policies, priorities (such as for health care funding) and decisions (such as political decisions) that might affect them; and uses this knowledge to help develop a vision for the organization to guide its policies and planning. External awareness helps the leader develop their own vision by highlighting opportunities and helping to identify factors that might help or hinder progress on the way to achieving it. It provides the context for strategic thinking and is the key to the 'setting' component of transformational leadership.

It is equally essential for leadership developers to have good external awareness and to develop appropriate strategies to deal with issues in the external environment, if programs and projects are to be successful. A number of factors in a politically and economically unstable environment can help create uncertainty, even antagonism in people on a personal level and strategies must be developed to overcome these. Developers can use their knowledge of potential support and sponsorship sources to help overcome economic difficulties and can bring key people into negotiations when timely, to help deal with a number of other environmental issues. A developer's own commitment and motivation are also keys to success.

Timing is another important factor in external awareness as the following two comments indicate.

Timing

'In some cases significant organization-wide improvements . . . were registered [noted] where the environment was conducive to change, e.g. where there were strong external pressures for change.'[13] (East, Central and Southern Africa)

'One constraint on the impact of LFC™ was the varying extent to which public sector reform initiatives might have created an environment more sensitised to issues of quality of care and the need for effective leadership and management.'[14]

Sometimes there is a tendency to push ahead with initiatives without being fully aware of the 'readiness' of the environment to receive them, or insufficient preparation of the environment and people in it.

Influence

Influence is the ability to help change the thinking and behavior of others to achieve desired goals. It is the ability to help bring about change – in practice, in attitude, in policy and in law. It is the ability to help determine decisions and directions. It can involve the appropriate use of negotiation, authority, or persuasion, or it can mean convincing others through well-researched arguments, debates and proposals. Influencing others is using effective communication, networks and strategies to provide information and motivate others to change their thinking and behavior.

Influence

- 'I want to learn new strategies for maintaining enthusiasm because that attracts people . . .'[15] (Costa Rica)
- 'I am now better able to talk about controversial issues in a positive and succinct manner . . .'[16] (Jamaica)
- 'With the development of political capacity came more power to influence and ability to negotiate.'[17] (Argentina)
- 'Because our project re-established better relationships, improved communication and showed negotiation skills, there is now a more respectful attitude towards nursing from other health care providers . . . the image of nursing has improved . . . we have shown we can make positive changes . . . we learned how to motivate the higher authority, and senior officials are very happy with our results.'[18] (Bangladesh)

Motivation

Motivation involves having and demonstrating commitment and energy to working toward the vision and achieving goals and targets. It means being able to communicate the vision to others and enlist their support. It is being able to take people with you toward key goals. Motivating means generating in others an enthusiasm, commitment and sense of purpose toward shared goals, in such a way that others have both the desire and energy to help achieve these key goals. Motivation is having the will to succeed, and generating this in others. It is providing the inspiration.

Motivation

'A highlight of the project . . . was that others became motivated to make improvements.'[19] (Myanmar)

'What she has gained is enthusiasm. She will be the type to role model leadership to others.'[20] (Zambia)

Confidence

Confidence means having confidence in oneself and what one is doing, believing in the vision and making this belief clear and explicit to others. It involves making judgments and decisions in a way that gives other people confidence. Kanter[21] believes it is necessary to make the connection between whether people have confidence in their leader and the self-confidence of the leader. She believes that although many leaders have self-confidence, this is not the real secret of leadership. Rather, the more essential ingredient is whether they (the leaders) have confidence in other people and therefore can create the conditions in which the people they lead (the followers) can get the work done.

The following example describes the development of confidence of leaders in themselves and in others and of key stakeholders in the leaders, over a period of time where leadership development activities were sustained.

Confidence

Some earlier ICN LFC™ team projects were less successful than others, particularly where there was little involvement of key stakeholders and when team members did most of the work themselves. This probably reflected their own level of self-confidence and that they were not yet ready to have full confidence in others. Learning from this, strategies were implemented by participants in later programs, including:

● establishing Project Advisory Committees of key stakeholders
● involving a range of personnel in the projects
● marketing the project aims and strategies to the broader
● organization

(continued)

- getting support from key people
- planning ahead for transfer of ownership of the project at its completion by selecting the person or persons the teams had confidence in to continue with successful strategies and monitor outcomes to ensure there was no 'slippage' (especially with quality improvement projects)

With the implementation of the Training of Trainers (TOT) initiative, it has been rewarding to see how confidence has grown in the trainers. There have been further opportunities for them to develop and consolidate a range of skills during the process of 'living leadership' in challenging environments. Thus, in trainer-led LFC™ programs, we have witnessed growing confidence of these leaders in themselves and in others and confidence of key stakeholders in them. This has had many positive outcomes, not the least of which have been increasing the commitment of key stakeholders to nursing leadership development and obtaining financial sponsorship for future programs because of demonstrated successes.

In living the leadership experience many trainers have been through tough times. Political and economic settings have often been constantly changing, as have the holders of key stakeholder positions. Some have been the target of personal jealousies of others and of strongly opinionated people putting up barriers to program development. Some trainers have held strong opinions themselves. Overall, they have had to learn to deal with these situations and revise and adapt their leadership behaviours to different circumstances. Where strategies met with success, confidence (in different people and at different levels) continued to grow.[22]

Kanter[23] says that leadership involves motivating others toward achievement in a coherent direction, building confidence in others and delivering confidence at every level. This includes self-confidence, confidence in each other, confidence in the system and the confidence of external investors and the public that their support is warranted. By believing in other people they make it possible for others to believe in them.

What exactly is confidence? Kanter says it is the expectation of success.[24] It connects expectations and performance. It comes from experiencing one's strengths in action, and it grows with repeated experiences of success, because this makes it easier to use similar skills next time.

Self-confidence comes with success

In nearly all LFC™ programs across many countries, different settings and different cultures, self-confidence was most often expressed as the characteristic or element of leadership that grew most quickly with learning activities in work settings, such as planning and implementation of team projects which involved skills such as teamwork, communication and negotiation. The more success and positive feedback participants had with individual and team project activities, the more their personal confidence grew.[25]

Kanter[26] states there are three cornerstones of confidence: accountability, collaboration and initiative. Accountability is taking personal responsibility, seeing where one's responsibility lies, facing it squarely, admitting mistakes quickly and doing something about them. Collaboration is teamwork, because confidence grows when you can count on the people around you and when they feel they can count on you.

Collaboration brings success and confidence

'We established cooperation, coordination and collaboration with respective township authorities, health personnel, and township NGOs [nongovernmental organizations]. This was what created the successful results for our project.'[27] (Myanmar)

Initiative means there is permission and encouragement for people to take initiative, so they feel supported and that their actions can make a difference. In this way there is confidence in the system, in each other and in the leaders – remembering that leaders do not do it all by themselves. Kanter[28] further states that each of these three cornerstones give both a hard and a soft side to leadership, for example – accountability also means data and measurement and performance appraisal; collaboration also means structuring teams and building an organization where people move across boundaries; and initiative often requires formal programs to solicit ideas and reward people for their contributions.

Developing confidence

'Chairing a meeting with the Director of Health Services and other dignitaries was a wonderful opportunity for me – a thing I never thought I could ever do.'[29] (East, Central and Southern Africa)

'I now talk with more confidence and certainty . . . and give clear and specific explanations.'[30] (Latin America)

'We developed a "can-do" attitude and our confidence increased.'[31] (Myanmar)

Trust

When people are involved in planning and decisions that affect them, are clear about the strategies to achieve the goals, and see these to be appropriate, then they will trust the leader. Without trust in the leader, the ability for the leader to motivate others is extremely difficult if not impossible in some situations. Kouzes and Posner[32] believe that mutual respect is what sustains extraordinary efforts, so leaders create an atmosphere of trust and human dignity and strengthen others, making each person feel capable and powerful.[33]

Trust

'We had to learn to work together as a team . . . it was difficult but eventually very rewarding.'[34] (Bangladesh)

'The experience has been exciting even if sometimes frustrating . . . Getting nurses on board with the project has been challenging . . .'[35] (Caribbean)

'I do not agree with her way of working. She is very inclined to lose sight of the focus, and puts on pressure to impose her ideas. I always had the feeling that she had no use for my contributions. She gives me the impression she is about to drown in a teacup. . . . The same thing with the team leader. She constantly kept up the pressure to impose her will . . . it was very stressful.'[36] (Latin America)

This last example suggests a lack of mutual respect and trust which made it difficult to move forward and achieve the best outcomes.

Political skill

Political skill is a key attribute of leadership. It does not necessarily relate to the political system (sometimes called the big 'P'), but is a term often used to mean understanding and coping with different and often conflicting, goals, expectations, values, fears and behaviors of different people, groups and key stakeholders. Having political skill in this way (the small 'p') involves valuing diversity in the people around you, and understanding the connections between different events and the factors that influence them.

Political skill means being able to plan and initiate effective, creative, proactive and appropriate strategies for different situations. It is using and fostering networks and strategic alliances, and involving key people in strategies and decisions. Political skill involves negotiating effectively, and selecting and using the best mix of talent in a team to get things done, thereby empowering others to make decisions and take responsibility for their actions. It is about using other peoples' assistance and understanding their perspectives – 'Where they are coming from'. It is being able to appreciate there are different ways of doing things than one's own way, and being able to manage negative attitudes and people rather than dismissing them. Here are two examples of political skills – small 'p'.

Political skill (small 'p')

'She worked as a change agent, deciding who would be best to help make the change . . . they discussed the possibilities, eventually gaining acceptance with the nurses then the surgeons. Over a three month period she used negotiation skills to counter negativism.'[37] (Seychelles)

'Nurse leaders must forge effective networks . . . Very early into the project, alliances were formalised with key persons in nursing, the public sector, the private sector, the media and NGOs.'[38] (Barbados)

Sometimes political (with a big 'P') is important in leadership too. It is using the political system strategically to help achieve a goal. The following example from Venezuela has components of both small 'p' and big 'P' political skills.

Political skills (small 'p' and big 'P')

'I would like to share with you all the overwhelming happiness we are feeling at the recent passing of the law on professional nursing practice. This was a goal which Venezuelan nurses have been fighting to achieve for over 40 years and which has now been realized, thanks to hard and conscientious teamwork, but moreover to our strategic work and negotiations at high legislative levels in Venezuela, mainly in the National Assembly. A series of strategies were developed and applied, such as the management of relevant negotiations, good and effective communication between the association's legislative committee and the national assembly's subcommittee for health, in addition to political contacts, which were extremely useful in achieving the objective.

'In order to accomplish this vision (dream), we developed a plan of activities which was developed step by step:

- maintained constant contact with members of the various political camps
- obtained 20,000 signatures of support accompanied by a document sent to the National Assembly's board of directors
- organized gatherings of nurses at the doors of the assembly, requesting approval of that law
- held regional forums to discuss and raise awareness of the draft legislation
- constantly revised the draft legislation with advisors from the assembly's health and social development committee.'[39] (Venezuela)

This law will regulate nursing practice in Venezuela and will provide recognition from the Venezuelan national government to nursing as a profession, not only factually but also legally, granting it full rights to practice public and private nursing in Venezuela. The correspondent for this example identified the following learned skills that helped achieve the goal.

Learning political skills through leadership development

- 'Communication: a great deal of preparation is required in handling communication so that the message can reach the interested parties as clearly as possible and influence them;
- Negotiation: as well as handling the negotiation and marketing tools, one had to speak with many people from different sectors and schools of thinking; this helped us to convince people;
- Political skills: knowledge must be had of the political party in order to use, with a social criterion, the relevant and important points in a law on practice and its contribution to improving the people's health; this is to say seeking the wellbeing

(*continued*)

of the population as the ultimate aim of any State, government or institutional policy, making people see that there is a contribution to be made, that there is added value for society and entities providing healthcare services;

- Generally: the education and training [leadership development] was of paramount importance in grasping the various management and leadership topics; it enhanced [my] knowledge and helped me contribute to the achievement of a great, long-standing wish of Venezuelan nurses: to have a legal instrument regulating professional nursing practice in Venezuela;
- Moreover, the program gave a great deal of inspiration to persevere with the plans we developed, and to make our dream – "the law" – come true.'[40] (Venezuela)

Review, change and renewal of self and others

Organizations, social movements, projects and systems all need ongoing review to ensure they remain in tune with their changing environments. Renewal and change may be required, meaning responding to new influences and pressures as they emerge. This means that effective leaders are proactive, initiating changes and new strategies as needed. They are always looking for ways to improve their strategies and systems. They are creative and innovative, not afraid to try new ideas. This may mean taking risks, but effective leaders accept that this may be necessary, and if the strategy does not work they accept that as learning rather than a failure and seek new or different innovations to respond to external pressures and requirements. Leaders in situations of rapid or major change recognize the pressures this brings to individuals. They encourage people, celebrate achievements and give recognition to individual or team contributions.

Review and renewal also takes place on an individual level. This applies to leaders and others. Here are some strategies:

- *Mentoring* is key to review and renewal of leaders. Mentors encourage, debate, challenge and point the leader in the direction of new ideas, trends and literature.
- *Peer review* and *performance-based performance appraisal systems* can be used at all levels in an organization – or project or team – to encourage leaders and followers to think broadly and relate their performance to the vision and goals.
- *Retreats*, or a team taking time out from the work environment for a few days to reflect on progress, strategies and results, can be a review and renewal strategy that is equally beneficial to the organization and the individuals.
- *Formal and continuing education* is another essential tool for individual renewal and should impact their leadership and through this, on their organization.

The following strategies (with examples) have been used successfully.

Strategies for review and renewal

- Mentoring: 'Our group mentor is a robust and experienced leader in both management and politics, and is employed in local government. I was able to draw from his experience and wise counsel . . . I have been able to identify and observe those "male" management characteristics, beliefs and aspirations . . . and was able to adopt attitudes that gave me confidence as a nurse leader. I have benefited tremendously and am grateful for this opportunity and exposure.'[41] (Zimbabwe)
- Continuing education: A significant number of participants in ICN LFC™ programs have reported increased motivation for continued study. A number have embarked on degree programs at different levels. Some attend different workshops and seminars. Others enrol in programs to learn new skills, such as computer technology and specific areas of clinical practice. Most have taken on one or more people to mentor themselves, and report this generally to be a stimulating experience as well as continued learning for them. In some countries there has been an increase in nurses receiving approval from employers to attend university for a higher nursing degree or PhD degree in nursing or education. In one country, nurses who had completed the ICN LFC™ program were more often successful in gaining places for continued study than other nurses.[42]
- Peer review: This is an important part of the ICN LFC™ program, and is practiced in a number of different situations. The following example is from an interview with a senior official: 'They [LFC™ participants] have become very objective and analytical in their peer review and feedback skills since the first workshop. They started out shy and very nice with their feedback. Now they are bold and provide constructive criticism with ideas and solutions for implementation and evaluation. This is a major achievement.'[43] (Seychelles)

Teamwork, partnerships and alliances

Teamwork is a critical part of effective leadership. It integrates the components of leader, setting and followers by using a diverse range of skills and ideas, and ensuring effective collaboration with key stakeholders in different settings and environments. It invites participation and communication and helps focus people on the mission and key goals. In particular, it helps empower those who might otherwise feel powerless, or unimportant to the organization or to those 'in authority'. Teamwork means learning to work with others to achieve common goals. It is underpinned by a sense of shared destiny. It involves developing people, delegating authority, and empowering and enabling others by:

- listening to ideas
- encouraging active participation
- removing bureaucratic barriers
- giving people the tools to do the job
- removing obstacles that hinder team performance
- encouraging and supporting creativity and imagination.

Effective teamwork

'over time, a strong team spirit developed among the participants. Through teamwork, participants not only enhanced their knowledge, skills and abilities but became more highly motivated to improve their own management practices and training work in LFC™ . . . those individuals that participated most frequently and intensively in the projects, experienced the greatest changes in their motivation, capacity and performance.'[44] (East, Central and Southern Africa)

However, for some people in leadership positions, encouraging teamwork and enabling and empowering staff is difficult. This may be because these people fear letting go, losing control, or losing popularity. They may feel they cannot trust others to do the job. If this is so, we must ask if these people are truly leaders or if they are called leaders because they occupy positions and roles that give them positional power. There is a difference. Earlier reference has been made to Hesselbein[45] stating that leadership is not about position, but that 'dispersed leadership' is the leadership of the future where there is not *a* leader, not *the* leader, but that there are *many* leaders dispersing the responsibilities of leadership across the organization. This is made possible by effective teamwork.

The ability to collaborate, and form partnerships and strategic alliances, is a critical component of leadership. It enables sharing of new information and ideas. It allows different parties to work together toward a common goal from a greater position of strength than one person or group alone might have. It can raise visibility on issues. It requires flexibility in thinking and the ability to work effectively together. It brings different perspectives and skills to the development and implementation of effective strategies. It helps to share workload where there may not be sufficient resources.

Collaboration and strategic alliances

In the ICN LFC™ program, different countries took a different approach to collaboration and strategic alliances according to their own situation. For example, wide participation of different stakeholders at community level was a strategic, organized and successful feature of some LFC™ team projects in Myanmar. In some countries in Latin America, formal networks or strategic alliances were established between teaching, service and management. ICN and ECSACON (the East, Central and Southern Africa College of Nursing, involving 14 countries) developed a formal joint venture (JV) agreement to plan, implement and manage the LFC™ program for the ECSA region. This contributed to a high level of local ownership and better support for country participants than would otherwise have been possible. ICN and the Singapore Nurses' Association also had a formal JV agreement for LFC™ in Singapore.[46]

An entrepreneur shares her perspective on leadership with nurses

Some leaders are very articulate in summing up what it means to them to be a leader. In Singapore, the participants in the ICN LFC™ phase 2 (trainer-led) program visited a public-listed company where the chief executive officer (CEO), a woman, had built her company with very small start-up capital until it had, at the time of the visit, a market value of around S$1.2 billion with plants in two other countries besides Singapore. The nurses were very impressed with this dynamic woman. They asked her many questions, and summarized her ideas on the important characteristics of a successful leader as follows.

What one entrepreneur had to say about leadership

- Must have a clear vision and dare to dream
- Never give up, and continue to press on when even when you tumble
- See obstacles and difficulties as opportunities
- Be curious and think without (outside) a box
- Keep looking out for potential people and be willing to nurture them, provide and facilitate opportunities for every party to grow
- Teach the fishing skills, not only giving out the fish
- Challenge people for their ideas but accept and allow the differences among individuals
- Take responsibility to make decisions and be accountable for mistakes
- Always enjoy the learning processes that lead us to success or failure.[47] (Singapore)

Note the emphasis on 'followers' in the above. Note also the emphasis on self-responsibility and 'learning by doing' that helps develop self-esteem and confidence. Here it is expressed in a way relevant to the cultural context: 'teach the fishing skills, not only giving out the fish'.

Are there other key qualities or characteristics of leadership?

Yes, certainly. The above discussion on characteristics of leadership is meant to emphasize the most important characteristics, not limit one's thinking only to that framework. Different writers identify and discuss different 'lists', but most would probably agree that the elements described above, whatever labels or headings given to them, are keys to successful leadership. Depending on the situations they are writing about, some might emphasize different attributes, such as managing information and technology, building effective teams, or being a skilled communicator, all of which are implied or inherent in the above.

Bethel's *Qualities that Make You a Leader*[48] is one example of a 'list' that reflects many of the elements of leadership we have been discussing (Box 3.2).

An assessment tool of 16 characteristics and their descriptors has been used by ICN in their LFC™ program:[49]

- Vision and strategic thinking
- External awareness
- Customer orientation

Box 3.2 Elements of leadership (Bethel).[48]

- A mission that matters
- Big thinker
- High ethics
- Change master
- Sensitive
- Risk taker
- Decision maker
- Uses power wisely
- Communicates effectively
- A team-builder
- Courageous
- Committed

- Vision
- A magnet that attracts others
- Building trust with followers
- Creating the future
- Inspires loyalty
- Expands the possible
- Releases potential
- Masters influence
- Forges productive relationships
- Maximizes people potential
- Strengthens resolve
- The glue to success

- Political skill
- Motivation
- Confidence and trust
- Influence and negotiation
- Creativity
- Interpersonal skills
- Team building
- Oral communication
- Written communication
- Self-direction
- Decisiveness
- Problem solving
- Review and change

A specific form of assessment was used with the above, involving self-assessment and assessment of self by peers, leaders and followers. This is a tool to provide information as part of a development program, not a definition of leadership. Therefore it should not be mistaken as part of a 'traits-based' theory of leadership.

(1) *Customer satisfaction* is one characteristic in the above group. This is of course particularly relevant to leaders in health. It involves a focus on the patient/client/customer, rather than on self as a provider. It is orientating one's actions to doing the very best for them, in a way that meets their expectations and gives them 'satisfaction'. Here is a good illustration of this, related to nursing in a resource-poor country.

Customer satisfaction

'Someday I expect someone to care for me this way – smiling, reassuring, caring for people, being able to explain that, even though there are no drugs, etc., I am here for you.'[50] (Zambia)

(2) *Core competencies* is another way of focusing on and describing key skills of the leader. It is often used more in a management/leadership context. For example, the core competencies of the twenty-first century leader have been identified by Krueger Wilson and Porter-O'Grady[51] in their chapter 'Are your management skills obsolete?' They identify the core competencies as being:

- *Conceptual* competencies, such as systems thinking, and acclimatization to chaos.
- *Participation* competencies, such as involvement, empowerment and accountability.
- *Interpersonal* competencies, such as facilitation, coaching.
- *Leadership* competencies, such as relationship dynamics, transformational style, technical expertise.

The first three competencies could be included under the heading of leadership. However, it emphasizes the point made earlier, that leadership is a key component of management in many situations and settings.

(3) *Servant leadership* is an important characteristic. It puts service to the needs of others as a main goal of leadership. The concept was introduced in 1970,[52] and later became a major part of many leadership writings. One example of particular relevance to nursing is Bethel,[53] writing about professional associations. She uses this concept in relation to the leadership of the association and its 'servants', promoting the idea of servant leadership as a vital quality for professional association leaders. Servant leadership in this context can be described as a commitment to serving others, for example the members, but also staff and boards of directors.

(4) *Achieving balance* is another critical characteristic. The risk of burn-out in a high-stress environment of constant change puts many pressures on a leader. If leaders cannot control stress factors effectively in themselves, it can be more difficult for them to provide a stabilizing influence for staff and others. Therefore leaders must learn how to balance personal life and needs with business and professional demands. This recognizes the development of the more turbulent environment described in Chapter 1 and emphasizes the need to be able to cope with stress and conflicting demands.

(5) *Emphasis on human and personal qualities* receives more attention in current leadership literature. Leadership is often viewed in a model stressing learning, listening, coaching, experimenting and networking with other leaders. The ideas focus on personal attributes such as confidence, ability to earn trust and respect, having good listening skills, giving encouragement, empowering others, leading by example, networking, taking risks and developing others as leaders. This book highlights the importance of leadership attributes and behaviors and promotes 'action learning' programs as the way to develop effective leaders. Such programs can enhance human qualities and develop behavioral skills. This, together with a sound knowledge and understanding of leadership theory and practice, will help ensure that the leader is perceived by others to have personal credibility and is successful in representing their organization.

Box 3.3   Negative behaviors of people in leadership positions that can diminish personal credibility.

- Showing personal bias
- Keeping quiet; not speaking up in meetings and public forums
- Keeping one's thoughts to oneself when they would be better in the open
- Not being willing to share, especially information
- Unfriendly competition with other leaders
- Being judgmental
- Demonstrating that one feels inferior
- Being over-critical of others, i.e. not constructive criticism within a positive framework such as peer review
- Being dominating
- Not listening to others
- Not recognizing other peoples' achievements

However, personal credibility can be diminished by some negative behavior of people in leadership positions, such as those shown in Box 3.3.

We have all witnessed some of these and other negative behaviors. Some will lessen as confidence grows, or in the process of good mentoring and leadership development programs. Leadership developers should be equally alert to these types of behavior as well as to more positive leadership behaviors that demonstrate growth and development. It must be remembered that leadership development is ongoing; it requires self-discipline and a readiness to expose oneself to review by others and to act on the outcomes. Some leaders will display the positive characteristics of good leadership – vision, ability to motivate others and lead them toward a shared goal, creative and flexible thinking, the ability to engender confidence and trust and to change with changing times. But sometimes when leaders get into certain leadership positions they can allow the trappings of the position to influence their leadership behaviors (Box 3.4).

Sometimes this happens when leaders are busy, tired, beset by deadlines and under stress. It can be insidious and creep up on the leader without them realizing what is happening and how others' perception of them is changing. They

---

Box 3.4   Negative behaviors when people allow the 'trappings of the position' to take over.

- Power might make them autocratic and less willing to involve others
- Being in the center of 'what is going on' might make them less willing to share knowledge with others
- They may want to use other people's work, or get others to take on some of their responsibilities while keeping the credit to themselves
- They spend more time 'being important' than leading
- They sometime put more energy into maintaining the perceived status of their position, than acting in a proactive and creative way in doing what the position really needs. The result often is that needed outputs drop, and less important outputs increase

go from credible to less credible without seeing it for themselves. This is one reason why ongoing mentoring is so important for leaders. To reiterate the words of Peter Drucker quoted at the beginning of this chapter, 'charisma can in fact be the undoing of some leaders as it can make them inflexible, convinced of their own infallibility, unable to change.'[54] Drucker is clear on how he sees charisma. Other thoughts he has on leadership include:[55]

- Leadership is work.
- It is thinking through the organization's mission, defining it and establishing it clearly and visibly.
- The leader sets the goals, sets the priorities and sets and maintains standards.
- The leader makes compromises and is painfully aware he or she is not in control of the universe.
- The leader sees leadership as responsibility rather than rank or privilege.
- When things go wrong, leaders do not blame others – the leader is the one ultimately responsible.
- The leader is not afraid of strength in associates and subordinates – they encourage it.
- The gravest indictment for a leader is for the organization to collapse as soon as the leader leaves.
- The effective leader knows that the ultimate task of leadership is to create human energies and human vision.

So effective leadership is not just about knowledge. It is also about skills and behaviors. The leadership knowledge and competencies reviewed in this chapter show the emphasis on skills, attributes and behaviors. In a teaching-learning setting, these cannot be easily developed by didactic methods. They require some form of 'action learning' that provides an environment for students to develop leadership and management behaviors. That is why good leadership and management development programs usually incorporate a significant component of 'action learning' or 'learning by doing', as part of their methods. This will be explored further in Chapters 5 and 6.

Finally, it is reiterated that leadership is not a neat 'package', easily defined and able to be interpreted in most situations. In today's world the environment is often chaotic, with pressures and influences brought to bear that can try even the most confident and steadfast leader. Norton and Smythe suggest that leadership comes from change in a 'place of shakiness . . . where doubt and certainty are always in flux'.[56] In the next chapter this idea is explored further in relation to the setting of leadership and the followers, to broaden the concept and understanding of what it means to be a leader.

Exercises and discussion questions

(1) Identify the main leadership 'theories' outlined in this chapter, and what some of the advantages and disadvantages are of each.

(2) With one or more key leaders in your organization, discuss their perspective on leadership. Try to talk with a variety of leaders, for example, a 'top' leader, a clinical leader, a professional or workplace (union) leader. What do they consider to be more, or less, significant in their particular leadership roles?

(3) Compare these ideas (from Exercise 2) with your own perspective and ideas on leadership.

(4) Identify those leadership behaviors and skills that you think you need to develop/learn more about. Discuss you self-review with other leaders, or with a mentor and get their ideas on how they see your leadership or leadership potential.

References and notes

(1) Norton, A. and Smythe, L. (2005) *Not Just Another Book About Leadership*. Pre-publication draft, pp. 9–10. Quoted with permission of the authors.

(2) Ahn, M.J., Adamson, J.S. and Dornbusch, D. (2004) From leaders to leadership: managing change. *Journal of Leadership and Organizational Studies*, 10 (4), 112.

(3) Kouzes, J.M. and Posner, B.Z. quoted in Sashkin, M., Rosenbach, W. 'A new vision of leadership'. In: Rosenbach W.E. and Taylor R.L. (eds) (1998) *Contemporary Issues in Leadership*, 4th ed. Colorado: Westview Press, p. 67. See also Kouzes, J.M. and Posner, B.Z. (1995) *The Leadership Challenge*. San Francisco: Jossey-Bass, p. 318.

(4) Grossman, S.C. and Valiga, T.M. (2000) *The New Leadership Challenge: Creating the Future of Nursing*. Philadelphia: F.A. Davis Company, p. 15.

(5) Drucker, P. (1992) *Managing for the Future: The 1990s and Beyond*. New York: Truman Talley Books, p. 121.

(6) Kouzes, J.M. and Posner, B.Z. (1995) *The Leadership Challenge*. San Francisco: Jossey-Bass, p. 318.

(7) *Ibid.*

(8) Hesselbein, F. (2004) Leadership imperatives in an age of change and discontinuity. Paper presented at the New Zealand Institute of Management Conference, October, p. 6.

(9) Participant report (1998) from Tanzania on progress in the ECSACON/ICN LFC™ program. ICN, unpublished.

(10) Report (2005) on monitoring visit for ICN LFC™ TOT in Tanzania. ICN, unpublished.

(11) Participant report (1998) from Zimbabwe on progress in the ECSACON/ICN LFC™ program. ICN, unpublished.

(12) End-of program evaluation summary (2001) for ICN LFC™ Caribbean and Latin America Phase 2 (Spanish speaking participants). Geneva: ICN, unpublished evaluation data.

(13) East, Central and Southern Africa College of Nursing (ECSACON) (2003) *Report on Evaluation of the ECSA Leadership and Management Programme*. Arusha: ECSACON and the Commonwealth Regional Health Community Secretariat, p. iv.

(14) ICN (2002) (developed by James Buchan). *Impact and Sustainability of the Leadership For Change™ Project 1996–2000*. Geneva: ICN, p. 29.

(15) Participant comment (1999) from Costa Rica in report on progress in the ICN LFC™ program for Caribbean and Latin America Phase 2. ICN, unpublished.

(16) Participant comment in *Nursing in the Caribbean, a Story of Leadership* (2002). Publication prepared by Wendy Kitson-Piggott, ICN Regional Project Leader for the Caribbean team. ICN LFC™ publication.

(17) Participant comment (1997) from Argentina in program evaluation document, ICN LFC™ Latin America. ICN, unpublished.

(18) Participant comments (2004) in project reports, ICN LFC™ Bangladesh. ICN, unpublished.

(19) Team project report (2005) in the ICN LFC™ TOT for Myanmar. ICN, unpublished.

(20) Mentor comment (2001) on a LFC™ participant, reported in the *Country Case Study for Zambia*, a component of the ICN LFC™ evaluation, 2000–2001. Geneva: ICN unpublished.

(21) Kanter, R.S. (2005) Interview in *Leader to Leader*, Winter, p. 21.

(22) ICN LFC™ program documentation (1997–2005).

(23) Kanter, R.S. (2005) Interview in *Leader to Leader*, Winter, p. 24.

(24) *Ibid.*, p. 22.

(25) LFC™ documentation during workshops, and in post-workshop evaluations (1997–2001) and ICN monitoring visits and reports for ICN LFC™ TOT (2002–2005). Unpublished.

(26) Kanter, R.S. (2005) Interview in *Leader to Leader*, Winter, p. 22.

(27) Team project report and comments (2005) during presentation of projects to key stakeholders, ICN LFC™ TOT Myanmar. Unpublished.

(28) Kanter, R.S. (2005) Interview in *Leader to Leader*, Winter, p. 27.

(29) Comment (1999) in participant report on progress for the ECSACON/ ICN LFC™ program. ICN, unpublished.

(30) Comment in participant report on progress for the ICN LFC™ program Caribbean and Latin America Phase 2. ICN, unpublished.

(31) Team project report (2005) ICN LFC™ TOT Myanmar. Unpublished.

(32) Kouzes, J.M. and Posner, B.Z. (1995) *The Leadership Challenge*. San Francisco: Jossey-Bass.

(33) *Ibid.*, p. 318.

(34) Team project report (2004) ICN LFC™ TOT program for Bangladesh. Unpublished.

(35) Participant comment in *Nursing in the Caribbean, a Story of Leadership* (2002) Publication prepared by Wendy Kitson-Piggott, ICN Regional Project Leader for the Caribbean team. ICN LFC™ publication.

(36) Participant report (2000) on progress, ICN LFC™ Caribbean and Latin America Phase 2. Geneva: ICN, unpublished document.

(37) Report (2001) on *Country Case Study for the Seychelles*, a component of the ICN LFC™ evaluation, 2000–2001. Geneva: ICN unpublished.

(38) Participant comment in *Nursing in the Caribbean, a Story of Leadership* (2002) Publication prepared by Wendy Kitson-Piggott, ICN Regional Project Leader for the Caribbean team. ICN LFC™ publication.

(39) Letter (2005) to ICN consultant from ICN LFC™ participant, now Trainer in the ICN LFC™ TOT for Venezuela.

(40) *Ibid.*, further correspondence from Venezuela participant.

(41) Comment in participant's progress report for the ECSACON/ICN LFC™ program.

(42) ICN LFC™ program documentation (1996–2005).

(43) Report (2001) on *Country Case Study for the Seychelles*, a component of the ICN LFC™ evaluation, 2000–2001. ICN, unpublished.

(44) East, Central and Southern Africa College of Nursing (ECSACON) (2003) *Report on Evaluation of the ECSA Leadership and Management Programme*. Arusha: ECSACON and the Commonwealth Regional Health Community Secretariat, pp. 61–62.

(45) Hesselbein, F. (2004) *Leadership Imperatives in an Age of Change and Discontinuity*, Paper presented at the New Zealand Institute of Management Conference, October, p. 2.

(46) ICN LFC™ documentation (1996–2005). ICN, unpublished.

(47) Participant summary (2005) of some important learning points from a site visit in ICN LFC™ TOT Singapore, shared with others in the program and with the ICN Consultant monitoring the program. Unpublished.

(48) Bethel, S.M. (1990) *Making a Difference: 12 Qualities That Make You a Leader*. New York: Berkley Books, pp. 9–10, 12.

(49) ICN LFC™ resource material (1996–2002). ICN, unpublished.

(50) Report (2001) on Country Case Study for Zambia, a component of the ICN LFC™ evaluation, 2000–2001. ICN, unpublished.

(51) Krueger Wilson, C. and Porter-O'Grady, T. (1999) Are your management skills obsolete? In: *Leading the Revolution in Health Care: Advancing Systems, Igniting Performance*. Gaithersburg, MD: Aspen Publishers, p. 49.

(52) Greenleaf, R. in an essay called *The Servant as Leader*. Later, his ideas were developed further: Greenleaf, R. (1977) *Servant Leader* (1991, 2002), the Robert K. Greenleaf Center for Servant Leadership, Paulist Press. Other authors, many associated with Greenleaf or the Greenleaf Center, have published on this topic.

(53) Bethel, S.M. (1993) *Beyond Management to Leadership: Designing the 21st Century Association*. Foundation of the American Society of Association Executives.

(54) Drucker, P. (1992) *Managing for the Future: The 1990s and Beyond*. New York: Truman Talley Books, p. 120.

(55) *Ibid.*, pp. 120–122.

(56) Norton, A. and Smythe, L. (2005) *Not Just Another Book About Leadership*. Pre-publication draft, p. 41. Quoted with permission of the authors.

Chapter 4
About leadership: the setting and the followers

In Chapter 3 the idea was introduced that leadership has three integrated components – the leader, the setting (situation where leadership occurs, or environment), and the followers. A simple illustration (see Figure 3.1) was used, and one circle in that illustration was discussed – the person who is the leader. Now in this chapter the other two circles are explored – the setting and the followers – remembering always that leading is living in 'a territory of shakiness, where doubt and certainty are always in flux'.[1]

The setting (environment) of leadership

The emphasis on the many components, attributes and characteristics involved in leadership will vary with different leadership settings. Some 'settings', with particular reference to the health system, are: type of (health care) organization (existing or desired); a social movement; a project; a work setting such as a hospital unit or primary health care practice; the political and policy environment or an environment of change. Examples of these 'settings' help to clarify the terms:

- *Health care organizations*: relatively unchanging; dynamic and rapidly changing; product-led (such as in industry); service-led (such as a hospital); military; government funded or revenue earning.
- *Professional associations*: nurses' associations; medical associations.
- *Social movements* (these often impact on health care): civil rights movements; feminist movement; political movements; religious movements.
- *Projects*: a quality improvement project; planning and commissioning a new facility; a public relations campaign.

- *Work settings*: the situation generated by a particular leadership role such as head of a hospital; senior nurse leader in Ministry of Health; leader of a clinical team; unit supervisor in a hospital.
- *Political and policy environments*: Development of new policy in governments and governmental organizations and in nongovernmental organizations (NGOs) including a variety of voluntary agencies.
- *Changing settings*: transforming an organization; introducing new policies and practices.

Each of the different settings described above can have a quite different social climate. Cammock[2] believes that leaders and followers, and their shared purposes, are only part of the leadership system, and he emphasizes the fundamental importance of the social climate in bringing leaders and followers together. Each of these settings might also require a different leadership 'style' and behavior. The different 'settings' are discussed below, with more consideration given to those directly relevant to nurse leaders.

Health care organizations

Different organizational models and stages of organizational development require different types of manager. There are 'change managers' with a particular set of skills, who are brought in to bring about major change in an organization. They have the strong leadership skills necessary for transforming the organization. They are, in fact, leaders. Sometimes they only stay until the change job is done, then move on to a similar challenge in another organization. In contrast, a more stable organization may require a different kind of leader and processes and systems to sustain its growth and development.

However, there are common attributes of leaders in both models. Both kinds of leader need to have the ability to envision the future, to review changes and long-term trends in the environment, and to think strategically and creatively about how to keep the organization strong and effective.

The environment today is one of change. This may affect different organizations in different ways, and some more than others. Bureaucratic organizations can be relatively effective in a specific context, i.e. stable, nonchanging environments. However as we noted in Chapter 2, they have generally proved unable to respond effectively and quickly to the pressing challenges facing health organizations today. The tradition of bureaucratic management style is one that just does not fit today's world. Many health organizations still seem slow to recognize this.

A 'bureaucratic' organization is a model at one end of a continuum and is outlined in Box 4.1.

Compare this with the organizational model at the other end of the continuum. This organization is flexible, open and responsive to a changing environment. The leader/manager encourages staff to develop knowledge and skills to be more innovative and accountable; develops a positive organizational culture; is strategic; motivates staff toward organizational goals; sets and monitors performance

---

Box 4.1 Model of a bureaucratic organization that cannot readily respond to change.

A bureaucratic organization:

- is highly centralized
- has many layers and levels
- relies on supervisors
- promotes conformity to rules and procedures
- emphasizes structure not process
- has no visible vision or future orientation
- does not encourage flexibility, creativity, and independent thinking or new ways
- does encourage stability, conformity, and *status quo*
- often does not have open communication with staff and the community
- can be autocratic
- often relies on authority of the position and positional power
- has no strong client focus
- has no real focus on goal-oriented performance and results

---

targets; relies more on development of staff for performance than on rules; is a good communicator; and sets clear targets and expects results. This model of an effective organization, described in Box 4.2, is generally recognized as able to be much more responsive to its environment and to changing demands and pressures.

The change to this second organizational model is not a new concept – these ideas about effective organizations have been described in the literature for over a decade. However, some health systems still seem slow to change their management styles and practices. Even when restructuring of organizations takes place, there is often not adequate or relevant management training and leadership development to support it. In a number of countries, even after 'restructuring', old

---

Box 4.2 Model of an effective organization that is flexible, open, and responsive to a changing environment.

An effective 'modern' organization:

- has a clear vision and is future oriented
- is strategic, with activities based on clear goals and targets
- has explicit organizational values
- has effective leadership
- has a flatter structure, and fewer rules and procedures
- encourages innovation and independent thinking
- is performance and results oriented
- encourages individual accountability
- invites staff and community participation
- has open communication, both internal and external
- is externally focused and responsive to its environment
- has staff oriented to the goals of the organization, not just to their own jobs

---

managers sometimes move into new positions and roles with little change in skills and mind-set. Thus those organizations are in danger of perpetuating the same cycle of managerial issues discussed in Chapter 1, because they do not have effective leadership nor do they integrate leadership into their management.

To do this successfully requires a different organizational mind-set. It requires first of all strategic thinking – being future oriented and having a vision to strive for and focusing more on *why* we are doing it and not on *how* we are doing it. The organization and its staff are externally aware and they become goal driven, that is focused on ends and results rather than the means of keeping systems going. Change, when it is needed, is managed rather than avoided. Staff and clients are consulted and their ideas asked for and respected. Innovation is encouraged. Staff become a valued resource, and staff development programs draw out their potential so that they become skilled, self-motivated and self-directed, and above all accountable for their actions. Systems and procedures are more fluid. All this is both a product and a reflection of leadership at the top of the organization, and it becomes so integrated into the management style that the two concepts are intertwined.

However, clearly it is not only the person at the top who requires the attributes and skills of leadership, but people in different roles and at different levels of the organization. The organization must function effectively as a whole. The changing leadership style from the top is one that reflects a more flattened organizational pyramid. It is leading people rather than giving orders from the top and developing and supporting people so they can work more creatively, yet within a framework of clear accountability. Staff must be performance and goal focused, accountable, open in their communication, good team players and able to assume team leadership roles and work in teams, be self-directed and willing to take and show initiative – all attributes of effective leadership.

Two distinct models of organizations have been described above – the bureaucratic model and the results-driven and performance-based model of effective organizations adaptable to change. In reality, because of factors affecting country health systems globally, such as migration, information technology, and the high cost of health care, we do not often find these two opposing models in their pure state. Many health care organizations today are a mixture of the two models. Even in countries with the bureaucratic model (and they do exist in a large number of countries and in different cultures), nurses often express frustration and a desire to contribute to organizational changes that would allow more innovation and the development of sound leadership at all levels.

Many health organizations are in transition from bureaucratic models to the exciting, more effective type of organization outlined above. Transition often means that some features of both models will co-exist. Sometimes this is very positive, but it can also be counterproductive. Some countries have gone for a major and quick transition from one model to the other. This is often referred to as 'transformational change'. It has many benefits, as all the linking parts of the organizational structure and systems become integrated and consolidated. But quick transitions can also bring problems, such as trauma for staff and difficulties in getting the support of the public if they only see negative effects of change. The goals and positive gains can become blurred in some quick transitions. More importantly, there is often not the time to develop and consolidate the kind of organizational behavior, or 'culture' that is critical for effective organizations. To be able to think strategically, being empowered to be creative and try out new patterns of work, taking risks and learning to be accountable for one's actions, are not always behaviors that are learned quickly.

When positions and their functions change as part of transformational change in an organization, position holders may need to seek counseling and advice on new and expanded functions and responsibilities. Often these positions are re-advertised and open to competition. Sometimes positions are disbanded and the position holders made redundant. Other times the incumbents are re-appointed or others brought in on the basis of seniority, often with little or no preparation for the changed role. Recruiting people with the necessary talent is not always easy. It may be threatening to other people who hold power. Painful situations are sometimes created, which the leaders and others have to deal with. So we need to think carefully about how to prepare leaders for change and the kind of education and experiences they need to equip them for new roles.

Leadership in organizations that change

In Chapter 1, the Leadership For Change™ (LFC™) team from Samoa was quoted as saying 'It is a challenge to adapt to and perform in a new system that encourages risk-taking, creative innovations and new developments'. The type of organization they had been working in was a traditional government centralized bureaucracy. Then the government of the country instituted a broad set of economic reforms which included the health sector. The type of organization that was promoted was to be results driven and performance based, and reflect a more open and flexible way of working with less emphasis on rules and procedures and more on trying new ways of doing things – and focusing on performance and accountability. Thus, the nurse leaders had to change their approach themselves in tune with the organizational and politico/economic changes about them.[3] (Samoa)

Professional associations

Professional associations are very much a function of their external environment. For example, if professional associations are to influence health policy, they must understand the policy environment. If they are to respond to their members they must understand not only the makeup of their membership, but also the issues those members are facing. Bethel[4] describes the type of leadership required by professional organizations as servant leadership, meaning a commitment to serving others such as the members, staff and Boards of Directors of professional associations.

Among the leadership skills particularly relevant to professional organizations is the ability to form productive networks, partnerships and strategic alliances. For example, professional associations can find it beneficial to join together to press for desired change, or to oppose what is seen to be detrimental to the membership (the 'followers') and the public. A united front and a coordinated campaign can achieve outcomes that an association working alone may not be able to.

Similarly, professional associations might require a different 'style' of leader depending on factors such as its past history of leadership, or the key goals and priorities to be achieved. For example, a period of turbulent leadership that has created some internal tensions in the association may need to be followed with leaders who have particular skills in negotiation, communication and establishing effective interpersonal relationships. And an association needing to strengthen its relationship with other external agencies and organizations, or its position in society, will need leadership committed to and able to meet these objectives.

Professional associations function within a broader social and political environment, so the association leadership must have 'external awareness' as has been described in the previous chapter. External awareness guides the leaders in developing appropriate strategies for different, often conflicting, situations. Without this key leadership attribute the association's position in society can be severely weakened.

Social movements

Great social movements in history, such as civil rights movements, have often been characterized by charismatic leadership. These charismatic leaders have inspired and motivated others toward a clear vision by their power of speech and oratory, or by the dreams and values they espouse, or by their personal style, or by personal attributes such as dignity, charm and absolute resolution of purpose. Charismatic leaders who have led significant social movements are people such as Nelson Mandela and Martin Luther King. They inspired others to great effort and achievement in the face of often extreme adversity.

The feminist movement in the earlier years of the twentieth century was a social movement with strong, determined, and, again, often charismatic leaders. They wielded power by their actions and their ability to challenge and eventually change many established social mores – and laws – in the society. Often they inspired some, while attracting anger, ridicule and strong resistance from others in their environment. The interaction between feminist leaders and their environment tells a story where the leaders cannot be divorced from their environment and where the interplay between the two is what ultimately shaped the outcome.

Projects

Different kinds of project often need different kinds of leadership, or weighting of leadership attributes. Here are a few examples:

- A special public relations or marketing project will require the leadership skills of excellent oral and written communication, perhaps negotiation skills, certainly an awareness of the external environment and a clear vision of the future to help motivate and influence the target audience.

- A quality improvement project may require in particular the skills of team-work, and how to build effective partnerships and collaborate with the different staff or groups involved. The leader cannot 'go it alone', as often many different categories of personnel are involved:

Working through others

'I have learnt to work through others to achieve some goals.'[5] (Caribbean country)

- A project to plan and commission a new facility will require strong planning and management skills, but the project leader must also be able to think strategically about all facets of the project, such as bringing together the various components at the right time.

Perhaps above all, the ability to select and lead an effective team is the most critical to leading a successful project. Attributes of effective teamwork, such as communication, motivation and the ability to influence and negotiate with others, imply or assume interaction with others in the setting, or with followers.

In project work in health care organizations, however, positive results are not always sustained. This can be because of the organizational culture, or changes in project team membership with insufficient preparation of incoming team members, or because of resource issues. There are many possible reasons. The project leader needs to ensure that project planning and ongoing monitoring focus on careful assessment of environmental influences that might hinder activities, or conversely that might be used positively to move the project forward. Some of the tools described under 'external awareness' in Chapter 3 might help, such as SWOT analysis, environmental scanning, or an analysis of helps and hindrances in the environment, or setting.

Work settings

There is a myriad of different work settings in the health system alone. The leadership style of bureaucratic versus open, flexible organizations has been described above. Clinical settings in hospitals need effective teamwork, initiative and strong decision-making skills. In public health settings the ability to involve and relate to communities and community groups and organizations is essential. Readers are encouraged to review the section above on what leadership is and relate this to their own work setting in order to determine the particular leadership skills and attributes that are likely to be most valued.

Restructuring as a part of health service reform has had a big impact on nurse leader roles, so we will use this as an example of a how a changing work setting influences nursing leadership. Looking specifically at nursing leadership in the past decade, one of the biggest changes has been in the role of senior nurses in health organizations, particularly hospitals and ministries of health. This has been directly influenced by restructuring in the health system, often characterized by decentralization. In these instances – and there are many of them – the senior nurse leaders who were the head of operational management lines have found themselves either in radically different roles or sometimes out of a job altogether.

In some organizations nurses still have direct responsibility for leadership and management of nursing services, but often with a different focus. For example, there may be less focus on management of *staff* providing services, and more focus on *professional nursing* matters such as standards, quality, implementing and evaluating new models of care. Some nurses have become leaders of service areas. This happens when organizations restructure away from provider groups, such as 'nursing services', 'medical and allied services' and 'administration services', to product areas based around client services. Examples include mental health services, child health services, medical-surgical services and infection control services. All staff working in such a service come under the service manager. One model is to have a clinical manager or leader (usually medical) working alongside the service manager. Where these changes happen, the leaders/managers are ideally appointed for their leadership and management skills, not because of a specific health professional background or 'seniority'. Sometimes nurse leaders have a combination of responsibilities – for example, for both nursing services and for some other service or area of responsibility related to the organization as a whole, such as human resources management or quality improvement.

Nurses are being appointed as chief executives of health care organizations. Some move into policy positions. Some go into private practice or consultancies. The opportunities for involvement in general health management are increasing all the time. Nurses are preparing themselves for these opportunities through a variety of educational opportunities, for example, in leadership programs, in nursing management, in business management, in general health management or in public policy.

Despite these opportunities, some countries have seen a loss (real or perceived) in the influence of nursing in the health system. In some countries, top nurse leader positions and roles have been lost in organizations and in governments as part of health sector restructuring. Sometimes the role has changed with restructuring, but often nursing has not prepared its leaders effectively enough to develop the new roles.

Changing the structure of an organization is no guarantee that the desired outcomes will happen. The leader must also develop the relevant leadership behaviors and organizational culture at the same time. For example, if the organization decentralizes, the leadership has a responsibility to ensure the staff can behave in the way outlined in Box 4.3.

Changes in the organizational structure greatly affect the nursing structure and ways of working. Changes in organizational culture must be reflected in the culture of nursing. Nursing cannot operate outside of the mainstream.

During initial and often quite disruptive organizational change, the need for nurses in professional leadership positions is often not recognized by the new

> **Box 4.3 Behavior required in decentralized organizations.**
>
> Leaders in decentralized organizations must ensure the staff:
>
> - are (and *feel*) empowered to make decisions
> - receive appropriate training
> - understand the organization's vision, so they have a context for decisions
> - know the goals and targets they are expected to achieve
> - know and are driven by the organization's core values
> - give and receive appropriate information
> - are part of and contribute to performance measurement and monitoring

management . . . or by nurses themselves, who are used to operational line management where nurses manage nurses. In ministries of health, the role of the 'chief nurse' (however designated) usually becomes one of policy – contributing to national health policy, advising government on nursing and, often, taking a leadership role in assisting other nurse leaders in government-funded health organizations to develop their new roles.

One way of describing nurse leader roles commonly developing in 'transformed' or 'reformed' health organizations is by the terms *corporate* and *professional*. This helps us to 'fit' nursing leadership roles and positions into new structures in such a way that nursing can influence health planning, policy development, and resource management in both nursing and the broader health service. At the same time, nursing retains control over the nursing function, i.e. professional nursing practice and the implementation of standards.

In the *corporate* role, the nurse leader provides nursing input into management at the corporate level, i.e. top-level management that has the overview and accountability for functions relating to the whole organization. Examples of functions usually managed from the corporate level are strategic planning, policy development, resource allocation, human resource management, quality improvement, and organizational culture and development. The role requires nurse leaders to have the knowledge, experience, expertise and perspective gained as a nurse, which will enable them to make an effective contribution at the top level. This may be for a health provider organization, a district or region, or nationally in a government-funded health care system. Sometimes nurse leaders take on the overall responsibility for other corporate functions such as human resources management and quality management.

The *professional* role relates to providing leadership and advice to management on professional nursing functions. Examples of these functions are setting and monitoring nursing standards, professional development, nursing legal matters, ethical issues, developing new roles and models for nursing practice, nursing skill mix, nursing research and demonstrating effectiveness of nursing interventions. These nurse leaders have to be strong on *nursing* matters. This is different from managing *nurses* and their activities and personnel matters. Sometimes nurse leaders have been strong on managing *nurses*, but less strong on managing *nursing*. Some have had considerable difficulty in transitioning to new roles that require

---

Box 4.4 The nurse leader/manager as part of the top, or corporate, team.

- A chief executive nurse provides valued leadership
- Nurses are actively involved in decision-making at board and executive levels
- Nurses participate in strategic planning at the organizational level
- Nurses collaborate with other health professionals in setting care standards
- Nurses determine the standards of nursing practice
- Quality improvement activities are in place
- The potential impact of all decisions relative to nursing is analyzed
- Nurses actively participate in the selection and assessment of technologies
- Nurses contribute to the development of computerized information systems
- Nurses have a key say in resource utilization
- Nurses shape their own staff development and professional education
- The organization fosters and supports nursing linkages with educational institutions

---

more emphasis on the latter. They may not have had the kind of education to support them in the new roles. On the other hand, some nurse leaders have had a broader education and experience relating to both professional nursing and to business skills, such as those required at the corporate level. Such nurse leaders have adapted more readily to the new roles that have developed.

The balance of corporate and professional functions will vary according to the organization, its primary purpose and the nature of the health care system. Some nurse leader roles are mainly related to nursing and to ensuring efficient, effective and high-quality nursing services. They do not include responsibilities for corporate management functions for the organization as a whole. But they operate at corporate level in the organization, meaning the nurse leader/manager is part of the top team, contributes to corporate management and usually reports directly to the chief executive. A decade ago a useful description of this role was advanced by the Canadian Nurses Association.[6] It is still relevant today as outlined in Box 4.4, particularly in those countries where restructuring and changed nurse leader roles are still emerging.

Take the following example which is based on a needs assessment to determine the key leadership and management needs of nurse leaders in order to improve management capacity. Note the emphasis on strategic thinking and planning.

Developing top nurse leader/managers

Nurse participants in one project in the Vietnam International Council of Nurses (ICN) LFC™ program focused on improving management capacity for district level chief nurses in four provinces of Vietnam, to better prepare them for their roles. The team surveyed 49 chief nurses at the district level to determine leadership and management learning needs. The priority educational need cited most frequently was strategic thinking and planning. The team then worked with the Ministry of Health to develop three training and development workshops for the 49 chief nurses.[7] (Vietnam)

But it is not only the senior nurses who are affected by the work setting, especially in times of major change. Outward migration of nurses is a major issue for many countries, further contributing to issues in the work setting such as conditions of work, staff shortages and difficulties in providing quality care. Some countries have seen leadership development programs, in-country and/or specific to an organization, as one way of trying to retain nurses and potential nurse leaders in the country.

Leadership development to counter outward migration

'Leadership development is one way to help counter outward migration. The Minister of Health and the NNA [national nurses' association] see the LFC™ program as an opportunity to give selected nurses advanced training in leadership and management. They said one of the greatest issues along with the migration of nurses is the lack of prepared leadership in the nursing profession in the nation.'[8] (St. Lucia)

Nurse leaders can also learn from other settings or work environments and be motivated to implement ideas of their own. This is one of the major values in leadership development, of study tours to other countries or planned experiences in other organizations.

Leaders learn from visits to other organizations

The ICN LFC™ plans, wherever possible, that participants make site visits to other organizations to learn and observe different aspects of leadership and management from them. Here are two examples:[9]

- In the East, Central and Southern Africa program the final workshop was held in Mauritius. The host country participants planned an excellent visit to a major luxury hotel to learn how the concept of customer satisfaction permeates all functions and activities in that setting. This visit motivated many of the participants to initiate quality improvement programs in their own settings, with a strong focus on customer satisfaction. (East, Central and Southern Africa)
- In Vietnam, participants made a site visit to a major hospital facility on the way to Ha Long Bay . . . many had never seen such a great facility in their country . . . they loved the experience and said it gave them the desire to go back as the head of their regions and hospitals to try to make changes that would make a difference in their own facilities. (Vietnam)

So, the work setting, or environment, can make a difference to the leader by motivating or de-motivating them, or by helping or hindering leadership activities. Conversely, the leader can make a difference to the work setting by being aware of potential issues and constraints as well as potential 'helps', and by implementing appropriate strategies, taking all environmental factors into account.

Political and policy environments

In some countries, nurses – individually or collectively – contribute significantly to regional or national health policy through their role or position, for example individually as the focal point for nursing in government, or collectively through a national nurses' association. In other instances some nurses move into positions entirely related to the development of health policy. They are often attached to health program areas in governments and governmental organizations and in non-governmental organizations, including a variety of voluntary agencies. They bring to these positions the background, experience and the knowledge they have gained through nursing.

Health is political. It commands a large share of government resources in most countries. It is a political issue even in countries where health insurance is the primary funding model. The following examples describe the interrelationships between the political environment, health and nursing.

Changes in the policy environment affect health and nursing

'Over the four year period of the LFC™ project, there has been a climate of instability in the health sector. There have been several changes at the political and health decision-making level . . . the climate among nurses has also been unsettled with a significant level of industrial action occurring and with a notable and increasing outward migration of nurses from here as well as from other Caribbean countries . . . there is rising public concern about key communicable and chronic diseases. Health and health services are thus very much on the national agenda. There was also reportedly a strongly bureaucratic public sector culture, including hierarchical management, risk-avoidance, and some resistance to change.

'The structure and strategies of the ICN LFC™ program challenged the existing norms. These contextual and environmental factors both helped and hindered LFC™ project progress and achievements. Public sector reform discussions and initiatives created an environment more sensitized to issues of quality care and the need for effective leadership and management. The most impressive impact was among the nursing stakeholders, both direct and indirect beneficiaries. There was a sense of empowerment and motivation among nurses interviewed, in spite of the feeling that health reform was at a standstill in hospitals. There was a general willingness to venture into areas that they would normally avoid, such as advocating for client needs, presentations on health issues and pursuit of nursing degrees. Several credited their new-found "courage" to the training, role-modeling and encouragement of LFC™ participants. The young nurses interviewed were very vocal and already challenging the status quo and had in fact begun to influence some changes at service delivery level.'[10] (Caribbean country)

'The LFC™ program has created significant impacts at individual and organizational levels. For instance, participants at the beginning of the program were not confident and could not articulate policy development issues during health sector reform but now they have acquired requisite knowledge and skills and are more proactive than before. Their presentation skills have greatly improved to influence creation of enabling policies.'[11] (East, Central and Southern Africa)

Box 4.5   Issues that hold nurses and nurse leaders back from being active in policy.

- The image others hold of nurses as a group
- The image that nurses have of themselves
- Conflicts with the woman's role (e.g. working hours)
- Difficulties in describing the value of nursing
- Inadequate education and political sensitization
- Nursing not making itself more visible
- Nursing not being sufficiently strategic in preparing itself
- Not realizing our (nurses') tremendous political power, or choosing not to use it
- Insufficient preparation for leadership roles

As health is expensive, the allocation of resources often becomes a very political decision. Nurse leaders should be involved in influencing health policy and political decisions, such as the allocation of health resources and priorities for spending. This is an important part of leadership. However the contribution of nursing is often invisible in the planning and organizing of health care services in some countries. And while it has the potential to be a strong political force, it has not systematically applied itself to influencing decision-making, and shaping health and social services. In particular, the role of nurse leaders in government departments and ministries of health is critical. They have access to government officials and to the political system and have a major potential for impact on national policy.

Many countries have lost such positions as a result of health system reform changes, sometimes because their potential role in policy, as opposed to operational management, is not well understood by themselves, or others. Therefore development of leadership skills is a major priority for top-level nurse leaders in health systems undergoing major change. This applies to nurse leaders in government and health care organizations and also to those in professional nursing organizations. They should be actively engaged in the political process, seeking to influence politicians and policy, and advocating for social and health improvements for the population.

A number of issues hold nursing and nurse leaders back from being active in policy (Box 4.5).[12]

To strengthen participation in policy there are several useful strategies:[13]

- using power effectively
- developing informed positions and using them effectively
- education and development
- being accountable
- understanding gender implications
- marketing the benefits accurately
- articulating the value of nursing to others
- using formal and informal processes and systems
- forming and using strategic alliances

- selecting effective strategies for different situations
- appreciating the uses of both unity and diversity.

Short explanations of each of the above follow.

- *Using power effectively*. Nursing at both individual and collective level needs to develop a greater awareness and understanding of the nature of power, what power they have or could have, and how to use it effectively. Power should not be avoided or rejected, nor must it be misused. If we understand power better and have confidence in our knowledge, we can learn to use it more effectively. This requires education at all levels.
- *Developing informed positions and using them effectively*. A powerful position (or role) does not guarantee influence. That depends on the leadership qualities of the person in the position or role. Nursing must develop informed positions on key policy issues, market these strategically and position itself to make effective contributions in the policy arena, e.g. by holding key positions in government and by being represented on policy committees.
- *Education and development*. This includes general education, training in specific skills and preparation in other ways for assuming a key role in contributing to health and social policy. Contributing to health policy development is an integral part of the profession. Preparing nurses for policy participation and leadership should be seen as part of nursing practice and nursing education. Some nurses' associations may need to show more national leadership, develop greater vision in relation to their role in the political arena and be active in promoting the need for education and preparation in policy and (where relevant to the country situation) politics. This can be done through training, marketing the desired image of nursing, and helping nurses and nurses' associations believe they are (and must be) political.
- *Being accountable* (or *'It's up to us'*). Nursing should not 'blame' others or the policy environment for nonparticipation, or lack of visibility. It should exercise influence through its leadership and seek opportunities rather than see threats. It must be proactive, rather than passive or even apathetic. It must develop strategies for addressing difficulties. Above all, nursing should have pride in itself and the contribution it can make. Confidence and self-esteem (critical components of leadership as we have seen) are essential for progress. If we want change, we must be part of that change and not hold back when we have an important contribution to make.
- *Understanding gender implications*. The relationship of gender to the level of nursing participation in policy should be explored. This includes the positive benefits of a largely female profession, for example, through its ability to exert influence at community and municipal level. The 'negatives' are important too, such as time and role conflicts and the undervaluing of nursing by some groups as well as by many nurses themselves, because of the value placed on the position of nursing and women in society.
- *Marketing the benefits accurately*. It is necessary to interpret the benefits of nursing participation in policy, to society, the public and the health services.

Justifying nursing participation in terms of its benefits to nurses, or nursing, is both ineffective and self-defeating. Altruism within nursing is sometimes misused.

- *Articulating the value of nursing to others.* The ability to articulate and demonstrate what nursing can contribute to policy and decision-making processes can help change the image of nursing in society with key groups and within nursing itself. It can enable entry into the process and ensure a nursing voice is heard. NNAs and other professional organizations should strengthen their statements on the value of nursing and the contribution it can make.
- *Using formal and informal processes and systems.* Policy involvement is not just through formal structures, such as holding office at a municipal or national level. It is also integrated into our day-to-day activities in nursing, both individually and collectively.
- *Forming and using strategic alliances.* This is another important part of leadership and is essential for exerting a focused influence in policy and political decision-making processes. Alliances might be formed between NNAs/other organizations and politicians/political parties in countries where this is appropriate. Particularly important are alliances with other powerful nurses in society, and with other associations of health care professionals, or with community groups and organizations who have similar agendas and a major role in contributing their voice to policy and planning decisions.
- *Selecting effective strategies for different situations.* Learning and skills development for effective strategies, and how and when to use them, is essential. Among the important skills for nurses to acquire in relation to this are:
  - media skills
  - strategic timing
  - being articulate and being able to make effective presentations
  - researching and preparing presentations well
  - strengthening the role of NNAs/professional organizations and their position in society
  - forming partnerships and strategic alliances (see above)
  - participating in policy debates in both the health and social policy arenas.
- *Appreciating the uses of both unity and diversity.* Nursing is not homogeneous. There are very many different interest groups. It must learn both the importance of unity and the value of diversity. Teamwork, partnerships, coordination and inclusiveness are essential values to guide policy activities, while at the same time, using the uniqueness of different groups to the best advantage.

Some further strategies that individual nurse leaders and nursing professional associations can use to contribute to and influence health and social policy are outlined in Box 4.6.

Nursing leaders can influence health and social policy through their leadership roles, and many see the need to develop their skills in this area. Readers are also referred to the section on contributing to health policy in Chapter 10.

Box 4.6   Strategies for individuals and nursing professional associations to influence health policy.

Individual nurse leaders	Nursing professional associations
Keep up to date with developments and develop informed positions	Lobby government and policy making bodies
Write and publish to help influence opinion	Position the association as an expert resource to be consulted by others
Join special interest organizations and channel opinions through them	Be alert to, and act on, health and public issues
Know who the key players are and influence them	Learn the most effective strategies to use in different policy processes
Work with nurses in key nursing positions and networks	Form strategic alliances with other organizations with similar policy positions
Identify and influence nurses in key positions outside nursing	Ensure public and written statements are clear and professionally presented
Communicate your position by different means	Develop and use unified positions with other nursing organizations
	Educate association members on public issues
	Ensure that those who represent the association are articulate and well briefed
	Prepare younger nurses for leadership roles
	Establish constructive relationships with influential people

Changing work environments

Where leaders operate in an environment of significant change, or are trying to initiate and manage significant change, they need to understand the key principles of change management.

(1) Change involves not just changing the organization's structure, but using the processes and systems that will get the best results. The staff are needed to make the change work and must therefore understand the purpose and outcomes to be expected. If they do not, resistance to the change can be expected.

(2) Change is highly personal. Duck[14] says that for changes to occur in any organization, each individual must think, feel, or do something different. Even in large organizations, leaders must win their followers one by one. Change

involves people. For some it may involve human reactions such as pain, anger, fear, uncertainty and insecurity. But for others, change might mean excitement, challenge, or perceived opportunity. The effective leader managing change recognizes and 'manages' the human, personal factors, such as excellent communication, involving people in change that affects them, listening to concerns as well as to good ideas, supporting and encouraging people, and demonstrating a caring and responsible approach.

(3) Change should involve the people it most affects. If people understand the changes, and are part of the planning and implementation, there is more likely to be ownership and a greater degree of acceptance. The opposite also holds true – less involvement may mean less buy-in and, sometimes, active resistance. Involvement of staff also helps build a positive organizational culture. We have discussed the inclusion of both leaders and followers as being an essential part of leadership. So it is important to understand the 'follower' attributes that can be developed by effective change processes. These include empowerment, accountability, effective decision-making, innovation and creativity, confidence and team skills.

(4) Change should be supported from the top. An organization soon becomes aware of lack of real interest or commitment from the leader at the top. Why should staff put energy into change, if top management seems to take little ownership?

(5) Change should be linked to the organization's vision and strategic goals, so that people understand that the purpose of the change is to better move the organization toward its vision and its key goals.

(6) Change should be well managed by leaders who understand about change management and especially the importance of full participation in the change process.

The following finding emphasizes the importance of the environment in supporting change, regardless of the leadership qualities of the leaders themselves. It also reflects the six principles of change outlined above.

Importance of the environment (setting) in supporting change

'While individuals' motivation, capacity and performance were shown to be strong, they were not always able to influence organization-wide improvements. Where organization-wide changes did occur, the following were usually in place:

- the environment was conducive to change (e.g. strong external pressure)
- top managers provided adequate leadership for change
- a number of staff were involved in the change process and committed to it
- appropriate institutional innovations were made available or developed
- some resources were provided for change (e.g. dedicated time for key staff; sometimes budgets for training)
- there was adequate management of the change process.'[15] (East, Central and Southern Africa)

This helps illustrate why people who are leading in an environment of change must understand the change process. They must involve others and empower others to act to bring about changes and improvements. Consider the significant differences between the two countries in the following example.

> **Comparison of the role of the environment in change in two countries**
>
> In Country A there was lack of coordination and agreement among the critical players who tried to set the project into action. 'Every person and entity worked on their own, closing the space for others to participate . . . and even though the LFC™ participants were deeply motivated to promote and initiate change, such motivation did not extend to others.' However, in Country B, there was wide participation in the project. The work institutions gave people the needed time to participate. The key organizations involved worked together. All key actors and organizations were motivated to initiate the changes.[16] (Latin America)

The reasons why transformation change often fails have been identified by Kotter.[17] Among the reasons he cites are a lack of real vision or not communicating it and not empowering others to act on the vision. These are critical components of leadership. And Hesselbein describes leading change as the great leadership imperative, where the challenges will be exceeded only by opportunities to lead, to innovate, to change lives, to shape the future.[18]

The followers

Leader–follower interaction

Leadership involves leaders and followers interacting in particular social contexts.[19] Probably not enough attention has been given to the role of followers in effective leadership. They have an essential part to play in achieving the organization's outcomes. So followers need development too, to give them the confidence necessary to help achieve the outcomes for the organization.

Followers as well as leaders can be developed by mentoring and other forms of support. This can help align them to the goals of a project, or to an organization's vision and goals. It will help bring people together and focus effort on aspirations and aims held in common. This is highlighted below.

> **Mentors help develop followers**
>
> '. . . mentors reported that they had aided participants in project design, monitoring and evaluation, confidence at work, willingness to share experience, confidence to take initiatives, clearer vision, written and oral communication, feedback on work performance, and personal and professional development.'[20]

A transformational leader motivates followers. Followers then become high performers who share the leader's vision and can help transform it into action. This clearly implies an active, dynamic interrelationship between leaders and followers, with each dependent on the other if leadership is to be effective. It is reflected in the following example.

Followers help the organization move forward

'Staff became more motivated and committed to the organization. Changes were also beginning to emerge in the organizational culture toward greater participation, transparency, and an orientation to performance . . . there was reduced uncertainty, resulting from a demonstrated ability [of the nurse leader] to deal with external pressures and to manage change.'[21] (East, Central and Southern Africa)

The leader who tries to 'go it alone' is simply not a leader, however humbling it might be to appreciate this.

Thus followers are an integral part of leadership. They help to support the vision and by their actions make it possible to achieve it. They are not a compliant group, doing what they are told and following directions set by others. They cannot be dominated. They work with the leader in a mutually reinforcing role which, together with the setting in which they interact, is what makes leadership work. Cammock believes that in discussions on leadership, it is common practice to abstract the leader out of the social context that sustains or frustrates him or her, and to attribute success or failure entirely to the leader. 'In this romanticized and heroic view of leadership the critical role of followers is almost invariably underplayed.'[22]

So an environment needs to be established in which followers can take even small steps and believe that their small steps make a difference. They cannot wait for the big moves made by the leaders at the top, but must believe they are an important part of the system and that their contribution can – and does – make a difference. This way they build their confidence in the system, in their colleagues and in their leaders.

Developing the confidence of followers

'In Kenya, the LFC™ team project outcomes are published in the national peer-reviewed journal. This encourages them, and also gets results out to others.'[23] (Kenya)

There are also times when the leadership role will change from the hands of the formal leader, to those of the followers. At these times, the followers take on the leadership role in support of, or even instead of, the leader.[24]

So if these two roles are closely inter-related, how do we differentiate between them? Grossman and Valiga[25] identify the following differences.

Leaders:

- study and create new ideas
- make decisions
- assign responsibilities
- create environment of trust
- take risks
- are reliable
- are loyal to followers
- are self-confident
- assume leadership.

Followers:

- test new ideas
- challenge decisions
- accept responsibilities
- use freedom responsibly
- risk following
- are trustworthy and respectful
- are loyal to the leader
- know themselves well
- follow as appropriate.

Teamwork

Finally, a word about effective teamwork and involvement of followers. Learning to work with others to achieve common goals is critical in leadership. Many believe that the key to making a team strong is a sense of shared destiny.[26] This emphasizes the importance of shared vision and goals. Everywhere we have seen how having a sense of vision is basic to effective leadership. Think about teams you have worked in. What teams have been most or least effective, and why?

Developing a culture of effective teams has many implications for the leader. It means being able to not only develop teams and delegate authority, but also to empower and enable the team members. Enabling staff involves:

- listening to ideas
- encouraging active participation
- removing bureaucratic barriers
- giving people the tools to do the job
- removing obstacles that hinder team performance
- encouraging and supporting creativity and imagination
- not having to have all the answers yourself
- letting other people 'shine'.

For some managers with a more 'bureaucratic' experience, encouraging teamwork and enabling and empowering staff is difficult because it may mean fear of letting go, or losing control, or trusting others and then having things 'go wrong' or losing status and perhaps popularity.

So teams must be selected wisely. Selecting only people who think as you do will not encourage critical thinking and innovation. You may have to let chaos and structure exist side by side, because teams in a chaotic environment need to be flexible and ever changing. However, they also need structure and good, solid process to get the best outcomes possible. Think about your own experiences in working with teams, and ask yourself what has been difficult, what has made working together easier and what has helped develop a strong team. This will help build a good working relationship between colleagues, and between leaders and followers. This in turn will build effective leadership.

Exercises and discussion questions

(1) Using the attributes outlined near the beginning of this chapter, how would you rate the effectiveness of your organization? In what areas do you consider it could be better?

(2) With a group of nursing colleagues, discuss how nursing leadership is exerted in your organization. Do you all agree? Who are the nurse leaders, and what is the evidence of their leadership?

(3) What factors in your work (or professional) setting, or environment, influence the ways in which nursing leadership is 'practiced'? How?

(4) Consider the ways in which your professional association influences health policy in your organization, or region, or country. What strategies would help to strengthen this?

(5) How strong is leader–follower interaction in your work setting or professional association? Does this need strengthening? If so, write down the strategies that you think would strengthen this interaction and the role of followers.

References and notes

(1) Norton, A. and Smythe, L. (2005) *Not Just Another Book About Leadership*, p. 41. Pre-publication draft.

(2) Cammock, P. (2003) *The Dance of Leadership: The Call for Soul in 21st Century Leadership.* Auckland: Prentice Hall Pearson Education in New Zealand Ltd., p. 13.

(3) Discussion and documentation (1997–1999) during the ICN LFC™ program for the Pacific.

(4) Bethel, S.M. (1993) *Beyond Management to Leadership: Designing the 21st Century Association.* Foundation of the American Society of Association Executives.

(5) Participant comment (1999) in program evaluation from the ICN LFC™ Caribbean. ICN, unpublished program evaluation data.

(6) Haines, J. (1993) *Leading in a Time of Change.* Ottawa: Canadian Nurses Association, pp. ii–iii.

(7) Report (2004) after the third workshop in the ICN LFC™ program for Vietnam. ICN, unpublished.

(8) Report (2005) on monitoring visit to St Lucia for the ICN LFC™ TOT, 2005. ICN, unpublished.

(9) Consultant experiences and observations during ICN LFC™ program implementation.

(10) Report (2001) on a country case study in the Caribbean, a component of the ICN LFC™ evaluation, 2000–2001. ICN, unpublished.

(11) East, Central and Southern Africa College of Nursing (ECSACON) (2003) *Report on Evaluation of the ECSA Leadership and Management Programme*. Arusha: ECSACON and the Commonwealth Regional Health Community Secretariat, p. 57.

(12) Based on the discussion forum (2001) *Influencing Health Policy*, held during the ICN Council of National Representatives meeting, Copenhagen.

(13) ICN (2005) *Health Policy Package*. Geneva: ICN.

(14) Duck, J.D. (1993) Managing change – the art of balancing. *Harvard Business Review*, 71(6), 109–118.

(15) East, Central and Southern Africa College of Nursing (ECSACON) (2003) *Report on Evaluation of the ECSA Leadership and Management Programme*. Arusha: ECSACON and the Commonwealth Regional Health Community Secretariat, pp. 58–59.

(16) Report on two *County Case Studies in Latin America*, a component of the ICN LFC™ evaluation, 2000–2001. ICN, unpublished.

(17) Kotter, J.P. (1995) Leading change: why transformation efforts fail. *Harvard Business Review,* March-April.

(18) Hesselbein, F. (2004) *Leadership Imperatives in an Age of Change and Discontinuity*, Paper presented at the New Zealand Institute of Management Conference, October.

(19) Cammock, P. (2003) *The Dance of Leadership*: *The Call for Soul in 21st Century Leadership*. Auckland: Prentice Hall Pearson Education in New Zealand Ltd., p. 27.

(20) ICN (2002) (developed by James Buchan). Impact and Sustainability of the Leadership For Change™ Project 1996–2000. Geneva: ICN, p. 32.

(21) East, Central and Southern Africa College of Nursing (ECSACON) (2003) *Report on Evaluation of the ECSA Leadership and Management Programme*. Arusha: ECSACON and the Commonwealth Regional Health Community Secretariat, pp. 51–52.

(22) Cammock, P. (2003) *The Dance of Leadership*: *The Call for Soul in 21st Century Leadership*. Auckland: Prentice Hall Pearson Education in New Zealand Ltd., p. 11.

(23) Report (2005) on monitoring visit for ICN LFC™ TOT in Kenya. ICN, unpublished.

(24) Cammock, P. (2003) *The Dance of Leadership*: *The Call for Soul in 21st Century Leadership*. Auckland: Prentice Hall Pearson Education in New Zealand Ltd., p. 13.

(25) Grossman, S.C. and Valiga, T.M. (2000) *The New Leadership Challenge: Creating the Future of Nursing*. Philadelphia: F.A. Davis Company, p. 52.

(26) Champy, J. (1995) *Re-engineering Management: the Mandate for New Leadership*. UK: Harper Collins.

Chapter 5
Developing leaders: designing a successful program

It follows that if leadership skills can be learned or developed, as asserted in Chapter 2, and the need for effective leadership is critical in changing and even in chaotic times, then it is no surprise that leadership development programs have flourished in some countries in recent years. Also not surprisingly, this appears to have occurred more in those countries where health and other types of organization and systems are attempting to come to grips with the challenges of their external environments – for example, public sector reform toward a focus on improved performance and greater efficiency. A range of different leadership development programs and opportunities are less of a feature of those countries still entrenched in fairly bureaucratic systems.

However, there is no argument that change in many facets of life is occurring rapidly across the world. Health systems are no exception, and change here is usually part of a broader economic restructuring. Nurses need to be part of these changes, and those who are or will be in key leadership and management positions need to be adequately prepared for new and expanded roles. They must have a good understanding of the context of their health systems, a vision of how health and nursing services may develop in their countries; the ability to plan strategically and to manage change; and the strength and confidence to

> **Box 5.1 Some characteristics of a successful leadership development program.**
>
> - The development of individual leadership characteristics and attributes that help make a person an effective leader in the broad sense of leadership as discussed in Chapters 3 and 4, taking account of the person who is the leader, the setting of leadership and the followers
> - The leaders will have a positive long-term impact in their professional and work environments
> - They will manage change effectively
> - The changes they initiate are able to be sustained in the longer term, or modified in a positive way in response to changes in the external environment
> - They will continue to focus on their own continuing development throughout their professional lives
> - They will actively encourage the development of others and emerging leaders

be proactive and fully involved in a challenging and often stressful change environment. Good leadership development programs can help make this happen.

This chapter is aimed more at those in policy or education who are responsible for planning and implementing leadership development programs.

What is a successful program?

Chapter 10 will discuss in more detail how we define 'success' in both leadership and leadership development. But a successful leadership development program should include at least the characteristics outlined in Box 5.1. These may seem rather lofty ambitions. Certainly not all leadership development programs will have this success 100% of the time. This does not mean the program is not successful – but if enough people emerge from a program with an ability to impact their sphere of influence, to sustain results they achieve and to influence key others, then the program could be said to be successful.

What is 'enough people'? Can that really be answered? It is useful to think in terms of a critical mass, which can vary in size in different countries, organizations, associations, or other settings. In this sense 'enough' means enough to motivate people to move toward a vision and key goals. Enough to:

- bring about improvements such as in the quality of health care
- help develop other leaders
- initiate and sustain new policies
- be able to share the leadership banner without succumbing to frustration, stress and the sheer hard work that may be involved.

All this implies that leadership development is not just about the individual, but about what difference they can make. That is the real measure of success.

Four keys to a program's success

There are four key areas that contribute to a program's success,[1] though not all the associated criteria will apply in every situation. The four keys are:

- Relevance
- Effectiveness
- Impact
- Sustainability

Relevance

- Linkages are established between the program and the environment within which the emerging leaders will operate, especially the stage of current or planned health sector change.
- Needs assessment takes account not only of the individual's development needs, but also of priority needs for the profession or type of organization or broad work setting they expect to operate in.
- Policy development and how to influence it is given high priority.
- Ongoing interaction between the program and key stakeholders is maintained.
- Monitoring and evaluation is ongoing to ensure changing needs are met and relevance assured.

Effectiveness

- Selection of people entering a program is critical: clear criteria are established and marketed.
- The program itself is marketed to key stakeholders.
- The focus is not only on individual development, but also on how individual leaders work with others in their settings to achieve sustainable innovation and relevant change.
- Effective teamwork is promoted as part of the program.
- Networking, partnerships and alliances with key stakeholders is stressed.
- Vision and strategic thinking is given a strong focus.
- Mentoring is an integral part of a program.
- An action-learning method is used.

Impact

- Buy-in and ownership by key stakeholders is essential.
- Alliances between the education provider (of the program) and health/other provider organizations will help ensure maximum impact.
- Systematic review, monitoring and feedback is provided for program participants and, where relevant, to their work setting.
- Project work associated with the program is meaningful and relevant to both participants and their expected work settings.

- Strategies are built into the program to help participants achieve successful outcomes in their work settings.

Sustainability

- People of influence with an interest in the outcomes of the program are involved from the beginning, to get commitment and support.
- Nurse leaders in the region commit their support.
- The goals and benefits of the program are marketed to key stakeholders.
- Key stakeholders are convinced of the benefits of the program.
- There is regular communication with and feedback to stakeholders.
- Younger people with potential are identified and brought into development programs.
- People already in leadership positions are also welcomed into development programs.
- Political influence is exerted where appropriate, to assist program funding and other resources, implementation and sustainability of results.
- Adequate resources are made available.
- Plans are made at program end for ongoing development and mentoring.
- Plans are made at program end for transfer of ownership of projects, where applicable, and for sustaining positive outcomes in individual development and organizational change.

Importance of involvement of key stakeholders

Running through the above is the recurring theme of excellent communication with and involvement of all key stakeholders (those who impact on or are impacted by specified activities and initiatives), right from the planning stage. Without this, program impact and sustainability of outcomes is severely weakened. It can make all the difference between *a* program and a *successful* program. Box 5.2 summarizes the most important points related to stakeholders.

In this example, important contributors to success are shared responsibility and accountability for different program components, shared resource mobilization and shared monitoring of progress. These can help generate a sense of shared 'ownership' of the program which in turn can lead to more effective marketing of both the program and its expected benefits in the organizations and countries concerned.

Other strategies to involve key stakeholders include different kinds of formal agreement and partnership (apart from joint ventures), working closely with program funders when there is no formal agreement, and establishing structures such as program advisory committees and program coordinators for specific situations.

Formal agreements provide a structured focus on involving key local stakeholders and can help in getting their commitment to the program. In addition, local networking is often strengthened. Similarly, advisory committees help

> **Box 5.2   The importance of stakeholders.**
>
> - For real impact, there needs to be 'ownership' by local stakeholders
> - The 'buy-in' of the main health providers, which in many countries includes the ministries of health and in others, university councils, is essential
> - Employers and supporting organizations must see the benefits to be derived for them
> - Coordination, communication and possibly formal alliances, with ministries of health and other health provider organizations, should be planned for, if it would help establish a formal advisory committee
> - There must be systematic program review and monitoring, with regular feedback to key stakeholders
> - The impact of program projects is greater if they are focused, well planned, involve others and are based on areas of need agreed with key organizations, such as employers, professional associations and different work settings
> - The individual commitment of nurse leaders and cooperation between them are essential
> - They are the key players in initiating and supporting other strategies and innovations to ensure an ongoing supply of well-prepared nurse leaders for a country or region

create 'buy-in' by key stakeholders, provide expert assistance and support, and help ensure that the programs meet identified needs and do not reflect only the opinions and perspectives of the provider of the program. It is partly for these reasons, and also partly for funding, that some business studies programs in universities enter into partnerships or agreements of some kind with local industry.

Program coordinators are needed when there must be a person *in loco parentis*, such as when the provider organization is in another city (as with distance learning programs) or in another country, as with International Council of Nurses Leadership for Change™ (ICN LFC™) and a number of other university leadership and management development programs. These people usually have responsibility for support, coaching and facilitation to ensure the smooth running of programs and to promote learning opportunities. They can monitor progress, keep all stakeholders advised of progress and issues and provide logistic support for program management. Thus it is important for key stakeholders to work together, and support and have a sense of ownership of programs, especially at local level. This can help ensure successful program outcomes.

So in all these areas – the important points relating to involvement of key stakeholders and promoting program success – it is worth investing time at the program planning stage. It may be too difficult to recover lost ground later, and any problem areas could grow. Later, in the implementation stage, program participants will take on much of this function as part of their learning and development. But it is the program manager's responsibility to make sure they get on the right track from the beginning and monitor ongoing progress and trends.

Marketing the program goals and expected benefits

It is also worth investing time in the development of good marketing materials and developing a marketing plan. But do not assume that because materials are sent out, people read them. Follow-up phone calls and often personal visits may be needed.

Marketing the goals and expected outcomes of the program should be done early on, before applications are sought. The information can also be sent out with application forms so people are clear on what the program is about. Give particular focus to employers, so they are clear about the benefits to them. Initial marketing is also often part of the process of seeking funding.

Some examples of marketing broad goals of a leadership development program for nurses are:

- To develop effective leaders who can:
  - influence policy
  - take leadership roles in health services and professional organizations
  - develop other future leaders
  - influence needed curricula change.
- To establish or increase networking among leaders.
- To improve quality and cost effectiveness in nursing and health services.
- To extend nursing's participation in, and contribution to, the broader health care team.

If you are not a nurse, and are reading this book, think about your own expectations of an effective leadership development program in your field. A variety of strategies should be used for marketing purposes, to extend the 'reach' and to attract the interest of different people in different positions or organizations.

> **Strategies to market team projects**
>
> In the East, Central and Southern Africa region, participant teams used a number of strategies to market their team projects. 'The main [marketing] activities undertaken were sensitization of key stakeholders; meetings; workshops; talks; presentations or sending of papers and reports; and the use of strategies such as the media, brochure distribution, newsletters and flyers.'[2] (East, Central and Southern Africa)

The other question to ask is how we can influence others to support, and perhaps fund, a leadership development program. Brochures can be developed to target potential funders, focusing on the benefits of the program. Different tools may be needed for key organizations and potential participants. Program beneficiaries, for example, could be:

- *Governments.* Governments often have a key role in health service provision within a broad socio-political and economic framework.
- *Policy makers and managers.* They design and implement health reform and other policies.

- *Health care providers.* They are at the sharp end of implementation and need to develop skills such as effective communication and good teamwork.
- *The public.* They are the recipients of health care delivery and benefit from quality care and improved access to services.
- *Other nurses.* They may receive a 'flow-on' effect from training, mentoring and other leadership development activities of leadership program participants.
- *Participants themselves.* They often receive a significant impact from leadership development programs and become more motivated towards achievement in an environment of change.

Box 5.3 gives a summary of the identified key *benefits* of the ICN LFC™.[3]

Material such as this, that is relevant to a specific program, can also be used for marketing purposes aimed at specific target audiences. In addition, an argument can be used for funders that they should support nurses, because nurses are known to be a key factor in balancing health service quality and cost effectiveness. This is of major importance in health care systems facing financial constraint. In addition, nurses are most often women, and women working with other women have a key influence on health in many countries. They often have excellent networks (for example, with nongovernmental organizations) and can influence and help in implementation of government policy related to health.

Designing the program: action learning

Many believe that the key to successful leadership development is action learning, or 'learning by doing'. With such a heavy behavioral weighting in leadership, especially in today's complex environments, how could it really be otherwise? The meaning of leadership was discussed in some detail in Chapters 3 and 4, and it was concluded that attributes and behaviors can be further developed, and new skills and behaviors can also be developed. Leaders can be made – they are not necessarily born that way. This view is supported by Posner and Kouzes[4] who showed that leadership is an observable, learnable set of practices. This belief is reflected in the action-learning leadership development programs that have appeared in many countries in more recent years.

Box 5.3   Benefits of a leadership development program that are useful for marketing purposes.

- Strong desire to be involved in health reform at national and local levels
- Determination to introduce changes at the workplace
- More effective participation in health teams
- Learning through networking and sharing with others
- Curriculum and teaching improvements for leadership development
- Improved partnerships and alliances with others
- Improved capacity in project planning, implementation and evaluation

---

Also essential in effective leadership development is getting the right balance between the three components of leadership outlined in Chapter 3, that is the leader, the setting and the followers. Leadership development that focuses only on developing the attributes of the individual has questionable value, unless it develops these attributes through practice and development opportunities in appropriate settings. This will also enable 'followers' to be part of the interaction in leadership development.

Successful leadership development involves person, setting and followers

'Respondents were asked to describe their most important achievements related to their country team projects . . . among these were obtaining stakeholder support, commitment and ownership; improvement in the quality of care; and implementing workshops [to develop others].'[5] (East, Central and Southern Africa)

'Participants acknowledged that project strategies allowed them to build on their existing potential and to develop new skills that supported their effectiveness as managers and leaders. Participants felt that their growth was in part due to the skills obtained in LFC™ training and to the implementation of the national project that allowed them to test these skills.'[6] (Barbados)

'We established rapport within the organization and with external organizations . . . developed skills to successfully motivate others . . . developed skill to successfully negotiate with higher authority.'[7] (Myanmar)

Many leadership development programs help organizations build up the 'critical mass' referred to earlier in this chapter as one of the factors helping to define success. This is helped by action learning which, by definition, requires the full and active participation of program participants. The degree of their commitment, motivation and self-direction helps determine the outcomes they achieve and the impact they subsequently have as leaders in their work setting and professional activities.

Many successful programs have some similar components. Each contributes in a different way to the total action-learning process, and interaction between the leader, setting and followers is integrated throughout. The common components are:

- structured teaching/learning, such as workshops, university programs and other
- team projects/syndicate group work
- individual and group learning activities
- mentoring
- formalized individual development planning.

Some leadership development programs have all of these components, while others have a combination such as mentoring, individual development planning, and some specific learning activities to enable development and sharpening of skills. In addition, where all components exist together, not all start and finish at the same time. Some may continue for years, such as mentoring and individual development planning. Other program content (such as session topics in structured teaching/learning settings, how mentors and coaches are selected and used, and group learning activities such as team projects or syndicate work, can be adapted to the learning needs of students. In fact, many programs emphasize working in teams ('learning sets', 'project teams', 'syndicates') and have at least some component of action learning built into the program.

Following is a brief comment on each of these five components, to help students, and their teachers and mentors, decide what might be more appropriate for their purpose.

- *Structured teaching/learning.* Often this is part of a university or other post-graduate program. Sometimes it is a series of workshops organized as part of an organization's continuing education program, or by a professional organization. It varies in content and length, depending on the type of program and student needs. If it is spaced over a reasonable period, it allows for ongoing action-learning activities (individual and group), mentoring and individual development planning to run concurrently.
- *Team projects/syndicate group work.* This is an important part of learning and development, and should also make a contribution to the student's employing/professional organization and to nursing and health services. Team members need to be easily accessible to each other to facilitate planning, communication and face-to-face meetings. For example, they can come from the same town, health provider area, or organization. It is useful if teams select the focus for their project in consultation with local stakeholders, and it is essential they gain the support of key stakeholders right from the beginning. Projects might involve developing a project plan in consultation with others, seeking funding and support, implementing the project (again involving others), monitoring progress, providing feedback and seeking advice from others and evaluation of the results. Progress can be reviewed at different stages in the structured teaching/learning settings through presentations and peer review.
- *Individual and group learning activities.* These should take place during the whole course of the leadership development program. They:
  - help students link content from reading and study to work and professional situations
  - help integrate the different components of a program
  - provide opportunities for action learning, practice and skill development
  - help sustain the development of leadership attributes and behaviors
  - involve and inform colleagues and others about their program and development, as well as team/syndicate group projects
  - help 'market' the value and potential contribution of nursing to the health services generally.

One type of learning activity that is usually very useful in linking formal program content to work and professional situations, is site visits to different types

> **Box 5.4   Examples of learning activities in a leadership development program.**
>
> - Delivering effective presentations
> - Speaking on a specified topic within a very short time frame so students develop confidence and learn to analyze and order their thoughts almost at the same time as they are speaking
> - Peer review sessions, to learn to give and receive feedback on performance
> - Team/syndicate project work
> - Negotiation and other role plays

of organization. This can also be a tool for raising the image of nursing in some situations. Here is one example of the value of site visits in a program in one country.[8]

Value of site visits to other organizations

'The Trainer has done a good job – she is a good example of thinking about creative ways to get the participants to stop thinking in a confined space, but rather to think and act broadly as well as locally. She took the participants on site visits. One was to a Regional Health Authority office where the issue of change management was the focus. The key points learned reinforced the "theory" of change management – but here they saw it in action and were able to discuss different aspects of it with the people actually involved. Change may be radical or incremental depending on the circumstance:

- understanding the organization culture is vital for success
- the value of communication, and communicating changes to staff
- performance targets must be realistic
- include the person affected in setting these targets
- a dominant strategy is training and cross-training
- the value of succession planning.

'Another site visit was to a large telephone company, where they focused on:

- customer service and employee development, which were discussed as key to organizational success
- strategies in the face of competition
- strategies used in preparing employees for organizational change
- forming partnerships.' (Jamaica)

Learning activities can cover a wide range depending on individual and group development needs. Examples are given in Box 5.4.

- *Mentoring.* Mentoring should be an integral part of leadership development programs, and mentor selection can be critical. Mentors coach and guide students, challenge their thinking and assist them with individual development planning. Mentors need not be nurses – it is more important for them to be effective leaders in their own fields, with the skills to help students develop and eventually become effective mentors themselves.

- *Formalized individual development planning.* This is entirely a participant responsibility. It assists students in planning how to meet their own development needs and career goals in a structured way. Mentors can guide and coach them and be a valuable resource. Students may also seek out other resources to assist them.

The art of mentoring

Mentoring has been identified as a critical part of leadership development, thus this concept is developed in more detail here. It can be extremely difficult to have a successful mentor–mentee relationship, as so much depends on the selection and skills of the mentor, and the motivation and commitment of both parties. The biggest challenges to successful mentoring are probably lack of time (perceived or real), lack of commitment and lack of clarity of the role. In addition, the 'chemistry' of the mentor–mentee relationship must be right if the relationship is to be successful, and both mentor and mentee need to learn how to terminate the relationship if it becomes nonproductive.

The following three examples from different parts of the Latin American region describe, first, a situation where a mentee had a nonproductive relationship which clearly she was unable to improve or bring to an end; second, a situation where the mentee kept her mentor but also found someone else she could relate to better; and third, a situation that the mentee gained clear benefits from.

Different mentoring outcomes within one region

'Contacts are not often, and are not very productive. I personally think that the relationship should have been done away with long ago'[9] (country in Central America)

'I worked with X on the IDP (Individual Development Plan). But where there were doubts on the project I consulted with Y who gave me all the information and guided me throughout . . . In part this was due to the incompatibility of criteria with X as I do not agree with her way of working . . . I submitted my final papers to her, on which she gave her opinion, but consultations on the process were with Y, who showed me cooperation and understanding'[10] (country in South America)

'Working with my mentor has strengthened my leadership capacity . . . we have discussed my weaker areas and I have developed confidence in change.'[11] (country in Central America)

A mentor is a person who agrees to take on protégés and to teach, guide, sponsor, validate, protect and communicate with them, in order to encourage their professional growth, development and sometimes advancement. Mentoring helps develop potential, capability, judgment and wisdom. Grossman and Valiga[12] describe a mentor as a close, trusted experienced counselor or guide who is accomplished and experienced, offers advice, and teaches, sponsors, and guides through significant points in their careers. They thus provide:

- counsel during times of stress
- encouragement during risk-taking endeavors
- intellectual challenges
- assistance in the development and enhancement of professional skills
- honest feedback, both positive and negative
- they see potential in people which the person may not see themselves.

So the mentor can be viewed as a career role model who actively advises, guides and promotes another person's career and training. They cultivate talent, take an interest in the person and are willing to facilitate their personal and professional growth. A mentor assists people to develop and use effective and appropriate networks. This is a very important function.

The mentee, or protégé, should be motivated, competent, dependable and interested. They must want to develop greater self-awareness, and they must want to exercise will.

Mentoring has positive outcomes for the protégé

'A number [of participants] reported an increase in confidence and self-esteem through being mentored, and an increase in knowledge because they were stimulated to read and learn more to keep abreast of developments, and to be good mentors themselves'[13] (East, Central and Southern Africa)

Peer relationships are important alternatives to conventional mentors, especially among top executives, including nurses. Both have the potential for providing support and sharing mutual concerns or plans, and ideas during change, including career change. Such relationships can at times be career enhancing. Some kind of mentor relationship is particularly important for top leaders and executives who might otherwise be in rather lonely positions. Effective leaders often have a mentor who helps expose their ideas to critical review and debate.

Mentor roles

Within the broad purpose of mentoring outlined above, several different roles can be identified. The emphasis will vary according to the individual mentoring relationship and the environment in which it takes place. The following adapted roles[14] are useful.

Communicator:

- encourages two-way exchange of ideas
- listens to career concerns and responds appropriately
- establishes an environment for open interaction
- schedules uninterrupted times for discussion
- acts as a sounding board for ideas and concerns.

Counselor:

- works with mentee to identify and understand career-related skills, interests and values
- helps evaluate career options
- helps plan strategies to achieve mutually agreed personal goals.

Coach:

- helps clarify performance goals and development needs
- teaches managerial and technical skills
- reinforces effective on-the-job performances
- recommends specific behaviors needing improvement
- clarifies and communicates organizational goals
- serves as role model for successful behaviors.

Advisor:

- communicates the formal and informal ways of progressing in the organization
- recommends beneficial training opportunities
- recommends strategies for career direction
- reviews individual development plan (IDP) regularly
- helps identify obstacles to career progression and appropriate action.

Broker:

- expands professional networks
- helps bring other 'learners' together for mutual assistance and benefit
- helps link mentee with educational and employment opportunities
- helps identify resources needed for career progression.

Referral agent:

- identifies resources to help mentee with specific problems
- follows these up to ensure they were useful.

Some people, rather than identifying different roles *within* mentoring, make a distinction between the role of mentor and coach. For example, one description of 'mentor' is that it is person focused, while the 'coach' is job focused. This seems consistent with the description of 'coach' in the above list. It is a useful distinction to consider when choosing a mentor. In addition, many people believe that an organizational culture that supports change and the improvement of performance, should also support an organizational mentoring system.

Responsibilities of an organizational mentor

Some of the key functions for mentors whose main purpose is to convey to a mentee, or protégé, the organization's culture, traditions, values and strategies for meeting the goals of the organization are given below.[15]

- Impart organizational skills
- Listen and question
- Show how to use the system to accomplish goals and specific competencies
- Praise and demonstrate trust
- Build confidence
- Encourage risk taking
- Provide counsel and support
- Act as a role model
- Assist in reaching goals
- Give constructive feedback
- Foster creativity
- Offer career advice
- Assist with self evaluation
- Provide networking opportunities
- Exhibit leadership
- Evaluate accomplishments
- Act as a companion, ally and co-learner

Mentee's responsibilities

The mentee has responsibilities too:[16]

- Willingness to accept constructive criticism
- Communicate
- Act professionally
- Exhibit flexibility
- Demonstrate initiative
- Notify mentor of problems or concerns
- Maintain confidentiality
- Express appreciation for the mentor's efforts
- Plan for personal well-being
- Be open to new ideas
- Respect the mentor's time
- Take action on the information provided by their mentor
- 'Pass on' the gift of mentoring (become a mentor)

Benefits

Mentoring should be mutually beneficial – both the mentor and the mentee should get something from the relationship. Applied in an organizational context, there should also be benefits for the organization. Here is an outline of the benefits for mentee, mentor and organization.[17]

For the mentee:

- learning new information
- gaining from the mentor's diverse skills and knowledge
- receiving advice and guidance on how to succeed
- understanding the organizational environment
- sharpening skills in handling stress, teaching and research
- enhancing self-esteem and personal growth
- receiving guidance on career transition across organizational lines.

For the mentor:

- opportunities to sharpen interpersonal and political skills
- satisfaction and fulfillment from helping colleagues
- recognition for improved job performance
- better staff skills, visibility and exposure
- staff commitment to the organization
- more effective line manager–subordinate relationships (if within the same organization).

For the organization:

- helps to deliver the vision and mission through achievement of goals and objectives
- increases staff performance and skills
- improves leadership effectiveness
- increases staff morale
- reduces staff absenteeism and attrition rate
- facilitates management's succession planning
- helps the organization identify performance deficiencies
- improves employee's insight about the organization.

Attributes of a good mentor

Some of the critical attributes of a good mentor are:

- *Credibility.* People who act as a mentor to another must be credible in their professional role or work position. They should be respected and well regarded by others.
- *Knowledge.* They should have a wide knowledge base. If their role is to include 'coaching' as a part of mentoring, then they should have a sound knowledge base related to key job functions and expected performance of the mentee.
- *Development skills.* These might include teaching, advising and professional development skills.
- *Vision.* Good mentors should have the ability to 'envision', or develop a picture of what the future might look like. This is essential, particularly if

they are to help the mentee to be forward looking in their career opportunities and in selecting appropriate strategies for personal and professional development.

- *High standards.* Mentors should set high standards for themselves and live by the standards they set. They should exhibit 'role model' behaviors that others will want to follow. They must also have an ability to encourage others to achieve high standards themselves.
- *The ability to challenge and debate.* Mentors must be able to challenge and debate ideas, decisions, skills, strengths, etc., of the person being mentored.
- *The ability to let the other person work things out for themselves.* This means not imposing ideas, giving advice too early, or providing the answers for the other person to adopt.

Choosing a mentor

Successful mentoring relationships do not happen by accident. People must make a careful and conscious effort to choose their mentor according to the qualities the proposed mentor has that will be most important to the mentee. To do this – to select on the basis of the qualities the mentor has – one must have sufficient self-awareness to know what is needed most. What career aspirations are there? What growth and development is needed? What changes in self does one need to make? A well-chosen mentor can help answer these questions.

> **Choosing a mentor**
>
> 'Before starting our project we recruited first a wise, experienced and cooperative-minded mentor.'[18] (Bangladesh)

It is useful to review the qualities required of successful mentors in three categories.[19]

- *Interpersonal skills.* Caring, encouraging, empathetic and nonjudgmental; able to help others develop a positive self-concept; communicates openly; can provide emotional support when needed; can be challenging and demanding and able to motivate others to high standards of performance.
- *Personal attributes.* Mature and wise, with a reputation for giving accurate and useful advice; friendly and has a positive outlook on life; admired and respected and considered to be both trustworthy and dependable.
- *Professional competencies.* Qualified and competent in their field, with the necessary experience to contribute to another; willing to share personal and professional experiences; has had experiences similar to those the mentee is now facing; has accurate and up-to-date information that can benefit a mentee; remains professionally involved and active in their profession; and is a person who continues to develop and learn.

This chapter has looked more at technical aspects of developing leaders, such as program design, program components (for example, mentoring and planned learning activities), marketing a program and working with key stake-holders. However, what Cammock[20] refers to as the soul of leadership has not yet been grasped. Cammock's concept of 'soul' was introduced in Chapter 2. He describes it as the emotion, identity and character of the leader that become important as they involve themselves in the leadership process. In the next chapter parts of this concept will be teased out as it relates to both leadership and to leadership development.

Exercises and discussion questions

(1) Review a leadership course, program, module (for example as part of a university degree) you have been involved in. Consider its effectiveness in relation to:
- Relevance
- Effectiveness
- Impact
- Sustainability

If you identify areas where any of the above could be improved, what strategies would you suggest? Write these down – it is a good exercise in analytical thinking.

(2) What components of 'action learning' did/does your leadership development program have? How were these helpful to you?
(3) Mentor relationships are an important part of leadership development. Review the part of this chapter that relates to mentoring. Is your mentor relationship effective for both the mentor and the mentee? Discuss with your mentor ways this relationship might be improved or strengthened.

References and notes

(1) Based on experience with the ICN LFC™ program, and reflected in discussions and available documentation on other leadership development programs.
(2) East, Central and Southern Africa College of Nursing (ECSACON) (2003) *Report on Evaluation of the ECSA Leadership and Management Programme*. Arusha: ECSACON and the Commonwealth Regional Health Community Secretariat, p. 38.
(3) ICN (2002) (developed by James Buchan). Impact and Sustainability of the Leadership For Change™ Project 1996–2000. Geneva: ICN, pp. 16–17.
(4) Posner, B.Z. and Kouzes, J.M. (1996) Ten lessons for leaders and leadership developers. *Journal of Leadership Studies*, 3(3), 3.
(5) East, Central and Southern Africa College of Nursing (ECSACON) (2003) *Report on Evaluation of the ECSA Leadership and Management Programme*. Arusha: ECSACON and the Commonwealth Regional Health Community Secretariat, p. 37.

(6) Report (2001) of *Country Case Study for Barbados*, a component of the ICN LFC™ evaluation, 2000–2001. ICN, unpublished.

(7) Team project report (2005) ICN LFC™ TOT Myanmar. Unpublished.

(8) Report (2005) on monitoring visit to Jamaica for ICN LFC™ TOT. ICN, unpublished.

(9) Participant report (1999) on progress, ICN LFC™ Phase 2 for Caribbean and Latin America. ICN, unpublished.

(10) Participant report (1999) on progress, ICN LFC™ Phase 2 for Caribbean and Latin America. ICN, unpublished.

(11) Participant comment (2000) in written evaluation, ICN LFC™ program for the Caribbean and Latin America Phase 2. ICN, unpublished evaluation data.

(12) Grossman, S.C. and Valiga, T.M. (2000) *The New Leadership Challenge: Creating the Future of Nursing.* Philadelphia: F.A. Davis Company, p. 199.

(13) East, Central and Southern Africa College of Nursing (ECSACON) (2003) *Report on Evaluation of the ECSA Leadership and Management Programme.* Arusha: ECSACON and the Commonwealth Regional Health Community Secretariat, p. 38.

(14) Geiger-DuMond, A.H. and Boyle, S.K. (1995) Mentoring: a practitioner's guide. *Training and Development,* 49(3), 52.

(15) University of Nebraska Cooperative Extension (2001) *Mentoring.* Lincoln: University of Nebraska.

(16) *Ibid.*

(17) Leong, M. *et al.* (2001) *Guidance Through Mentoring.* Booklet prepared by an SNA/ICN LFC™ Project Group. Singapore Nurses Association.

(18) Report (2004) on progress with team project, ICN LFC™ TOT program for Bangladesh. Unpublished.

(19) Appleby, D. (August 21, 2001) Choosing a Mentor. www.psichi.org/content/publications/eye/vol_3/3/applebyl.asp

(20) Cammock, P. (2003) *The Dance of Leadership: The Call for Soul in 21st Century Leadership.* Auckland: Prentice Hall Pearson Education in New Zealand Ltd.

Chapter 6
The 'soul' of leadership and leadership development

At the end of Chapter 5 it was asserted that leadership – and therefore leadership development – is enriched by 'soul'. Cammock's concept of the soul of leadership[1] is highlighted in Box 6.1.

This concept of 'soul' is now looked at in two ways. First in relation to the three-way concept of leadership that is used in this book, that is the person who is the leader, the setting of leadership and the followers. Second, in relation to a framework of ten 'lessons' described by Posner and Kouzes[2] based on their research, which showed them that leadership was an observable, learnable set of practices.

Leadership, leadership development and 'soul': person, setting and followers

How does 'emotion, identity and character' emerge during the leadership development process? Why is it important?

The person who is the leader

The person who is the leader is central to this concept. The leader must have the ability to inspire, motivate and influence. This may be with 'followers', or in the 'setting' with key stakeholders, with policy development, and with changes in systems and processes. A leadership development program can help inject 'soul',

---

Box 6.1   The concept of soul, as described by Cammock

Soul: The emotion, identity and character of the leader that become important as they involve themselves in the leadership process.

---

i.e. emotion, identity and character, into the person who is the leader, and also through this into the setting and the followers.

Putting 'soul' into leadership development

'The Trainer said that when she met the first group of participants they were fairly discouraged and de-motivated about everything . . . but she and her colleague challenged their thinking so much that they are now truly changed . . . I got to meet them at the beginning of the program and later as they were finishing up, and was impressed with the level of personal development they had achieved . . . we all went to the Opera House together and they were dressed for success, business cards, networking with all the NNA [national nurses' association] and other officials, Madame this, Mr. this and that . . . I would like . . . I am . . . I thought wow, at first this was a group of no energy, and now they are energized and proactive.'[3] (Jamaica)

An example of 'soul' often lies in the ability to envision and to be strategic – a key component of leadership. However, a program that 'teaches' the theory and practice of envisioning and strategic thinking will not necessarily inject 'soul' into the process. This takes more, and the answer can partly be found in related action-learning activities.

A team that develops and then acts on its own vision, such as for a nursing service, or for a specific project, will usually experience the 'lows' of frustration, or compromise on firmly held beliefs, or teamwork that is not always smooth. But it will also experience the 'highs' of satisfaction and ownership of the outcome, of confidence that it will help guide the team members themselves and others, of excitement about the future possibilities that it envisions, and of a sense of achievement when the team members see other peoples' action contribute to successful outcomes. They will *feel*. It will not be an empty exercise in the techniques of envisioning and strategic thinking, but a living, emotional experience. This emotion helps generate the team's ability to motivate and inspire others, and it helps to define the identity and character of the leader. It generates self-confidence and the ability to inspire confidence in others. Strategically chosen words written into vision statements can be powerful motivators too.

Take another example. Credibility and trust are important components of leadership and can grow during leadership development. Credibility of the leader comes when others recognize achievements and support the strategies and behaviors to achieve these.

Stakeholders recognize and support 'soul' in others

'They [local stakeholders] gave very positive comments on the teams' performance, especially their enthusiasm, initiative and effective communication with related authorities, nurses and supporting staff. The latter told that they also tried their best to provide co-operation and support.

(continued overleaf)

'Mentors and supervisors are interested to sustain the program. The authorities were requested to utilize the leadership skills acquired by the nurses and to provide the support and assistance to continue it. The team members were requested to think about future plans for project activities sustainability. Both stakeholders and team members emphasized the importance of follow-up monitoring visits.

'Places/wards under Project phase 1 were visited. In most of the places they had managed to sustain the same level of quality and enthusiasm, but due to shortage of supporting staff and transfer of higher authority, the team members reported some difficulties in some places . . . But generally there were highly motivated hospital authorities and unit team members. Team members are able to improve nursing image within the hospital environment towards their authorities and clients . . . Directors from the hospitals were satisfied in terms of clients' satisfaction and nurses' initiative for quality care.

'The hospital authorities were encouraging [them] to take similar initiatives in other wards. Even when constraints are there, the teams could successfully manage most of the problems. Throughout the project period, support and assistance from departments and authorities were excellent.'[4] (Bangladesh)

This example illustrates how credibility in nurse leaders can develop as a result of leadership development activities. The identity of nurses as leaders is enhanced. The image of nursing in the health service setting, the community, or the society is enhanced. The 'character' of leaders becomes defined in terms of attributes such as creativity in developing appropriate strategies, focused on outcomes and results, skilled in teamwork and the involvement of a variety of others to achieve their goals. Credibility leads to trust. Other people will provide support and are often 'enthusiastic' and 'highly motivated' as the above example shows.

In Chapter 3 it was suggested that trust in the leader develops if people are involved in planning and decisions that affect them, are clear about the strategies to achieve the goals and agree on the appropriateness of these. But without trust in the leader, the ability for the leader to motivate others is extremely difficult if not impossible in some situations. The following example shows how the developing leader, others in the setting and the 'followers', all developed some degree of trust because the project activities were perceived as credible.

Trust is developed through credible activities

Bangladesh is a resource-poor country where the ICN LFC™ [International Council of Nurses Leadership for Change™] has been implemented over five years (the first program was followed by programs implemented by Trainers under the LFC™ TOT [Training of Trainers] methodology). The foundation for credibility in the first program was laid during the envisioning process for team projects. Goals which may have seemed unachievable to themselves, stakeholders and colleagues, were governed by a vision that stated they were to be achieved 'within available resources'. Thus the scene

(continued)

was set for everyone to view the projects as possible within the reality of their situation, given creative strategies, negotiation skills and the ability to motivate and influence others. It generated excitement and satisfaction as key targets were achieved.

'A variety of key personnel within and outside nursing put their full weight and support behind the projects. Some hospital policies were changed. Strategies became incorporated in the newly normal way of doing things. The enthusiasm of the project teams helped convey a different image of nursing and what nursing leadership can be capable of. The soul of leadership development was at work. People were inspired. More importantly, credibility and trust were established and the groundwork of continued support from key stakeholders for ongoing leadership development programs was firmly laid.'[5] (Bangladesh)

Earlier Kouzes and Posner[6] were quoted regarding their belief that mutual respect is what sustains extraordinary efforts, where leaders create an atmosphere of trust and human dignity and strengthen others, making each person feel capable and powerful. There are instances of emotion here – part of the 'soul' of leadership. This too can be generated in leadership development programs that focus on learning by doing. Team projects or syndicate work are a significant and essential tool for the development not only of leadership skills and behaviors but also of the feelings, emotions and character of the leader that become integral to how that leader will operate in the future.

Where the 'soul' of leadership is more strongly developed, the person is more likely to sustain their development in the longer term. But where it is weaker, where lower commitment to the program and their own development is reflected in the way they go about their various learning activities, then sustained positive outcomes in terms of individual development is less likely. Sometimes this also reflects difficulties in the setting and with an apathetic and unmotivated follower group that the leader is not able to overcome by his or her efforts. Perhaps, in the words of Kouzes and Posner, there is insufficient mutual respect to sustain extraordinary efforts, as reflected in the following example.

Sustaining 'soul' in difficult environments (settings)

In one country where the ICN LFC™ was implemented, political and bureaucratic factors influenced the selection of participants. Some were selected on the basis of position and seniority, and had low commitment or motivation to their development. These (certainly not a majority) firmly believed that leadership is about position, which is a view discounted in this book in Chapter 2 (What leadership is not). Their contribution to project work was weak and the outcomes for them in terms if individual development were also weak. They were often critical of another group they considered 'too young', whereas this younger group did some excellent – and often far better – work.

But it was interesting to note that in most instances, the attitude of the 'positional' leaders did not necessarily detract from the development of other people in their teams.

(continued overleaf)

> In particular, where other participants were highly motivated and committed to
> longer-term changes in the nursing and health services, when they strongly (often
> expressed quite emotionally in the program environment) felt that things needed to
> change, then they focused on developing the skills and behaviors that they believed
> would contribute to that change in the future.
>
> Some of these people indicated that many 'followers' shared their vision for change.
> However, the 'setting' of political and government instability and influence on key
> appointments in the broader environment of this country, may well determine the extent
> to which the soul of leadership that some of these participants have clearly developed,
> is able to be sustained.[7]

The setting of leadership

The setting (situation or environment) of leadership is clearly significant to leadership development as it is to leadership itself. In Chapter 4 we discussed the
setting of leadership in terms of the organizations, professional associations, social
movements, projects, work settings, political and policy environments and
changing environments.

Leadership development programs that focus more on the individual and do not
take the influences of different settings into account, run grave risks of failure.
This failure can be in the individual, because of apathy or lack of support in
their work or country setting. It can be failure in terms of lack of successful
outcomes from projects, initiatives or other proposed changes in a work setting
that is relatively unchanging – even resistant to change. And it can be failure in
the work setting itself because of resistance, a strongly bureaucratic environment with few key people supporting the need to change, lack of credibility or
influence of the person who has undertaken the leadership development program,
insufficient or inadequate networking, lack of support or interest from key stakeholders and often absolute resistance to change. In fact, the more the setting leans
toward bureaucracy and bureaucratic management, the more difficult – though
not impossible – for the leader to influence sustainable changes in the work setting.

How can these potential failures be avoided? We suggest they hinge on the
'soul' of leadership development. In the setting or environment, this includes such
things as:

- *Empathy*: developing and demonstrating the capacity for empathy through
  working with a good mentor, through involving and listening to others in
  team projects, through effective networking and collaboration, and through
  acting on self- and peer-assessment of performance.
- *Excitement*: the 'glow of success' that comes from careful problem analysis
  and the development and implementation of strategies that produce effective
  outcomes. This can be developed through project work and other setting-
  related initiatives.
- *Encouragement*: encouragement of the developing leader through mentorship and through working with key stakeholders on team projects and other

learning activities. Through this the developing leader learns the value of supporting, developing and encouraging others.

- *Empowerment*: developing the right environment and helping others develop the skills that will help them achieve good results through their own actions. Through this they develop confidence in themselves and in a system that enables them to act, and where they can clearly see that their contribution makes a difference.

The importance of setting to 'soul' is highlighted in the following examples.

Facilitating 'soul' through the environment (setting)

Some key points related to the setting of leadership that help make a leadership development program more effective are:

- relevance to current or planned health sector change
- relevance to the priority needs of health systems and organizations
- commitment and support of key stakeholders and influential people
- commitment by nurse leaders
- cooperation between nurse leaders, particularly commitment from both national nurses' association and government chief nurse
- employers and supporting organizations are clear on the benefits.[8]

Where one or more of these factors are missing to a significant degree, then introducing 'soul' into leadership development becomes difficult. The risk of failure increases as the number and degree of the above factors decreases. Take the following examples from two small nations.

Setting can determine success or failure in developing 'soul'

In the first example, the timing was right as health sector change was on the agenda. The team project focused on a priority determined by the Ministry of Health, and the process and successful outcomes later became incorporated as policy. All key stakeholders supported the LFC™ program and participant learning activities. The Chief Nurse in government and the national nurses association worked closely together, with the former (a woman of immense credibility with all key stakeholders) acting as the mentor to program participants. Finally, the benefits of the program were clear to others and in fact other key people kept pace with and asked to share the learning from the program at each stage of its development. As a result the 'soul' of leadership development emerged: excitement and satisfaction from positive feedback, confidence in individual leadership skills and knowledge, pride in achievement, credibility and commitment to ongoing leadership development of others.

In the other example, the general nursing culture appeared to be one of apathy and there were no current plans for health sector change which would have added both stimulus and urgency to leadership development. A key nurse leader involved with

(*continued overleaf*)

both the government and the national nurses' association self-appointed herself as mentor. Criticism (of the developing leaders, the project and the program) was more apparent than was support and encouragement. Commitment from local stakeholders was low, partly because of the influence of the mentor. Instead of confidence and excitement emerging from a positive leadership development environment and positive outcomes from learning activities there was more apathy, lower self-esteem and little heart for further achievement. While other variables were no doubt operating in this situation, what is clear is that involvement in the LFC™ program in the absence of 'soul' in the work setting where so many of the learning activities took place, did not easily generate 'soul' in the person who was the developing leader.[9]

Those responsible for leadership development programs have as much responsibility to give attention to the setting as they do to the developing leaders. In some programs the setting is largely left to the developing leaders, for example communication with key stakeholders, fostering networking and partnerships, developing effective support systems, motivating and encouraging others and in turn receiving support and encouragement from mentors and stakeholders, and assessing and acting on environmental impacts. This is a key part of leadership development and responsibility must not be taken away from the developing leaders for this.

However, program directors also have a responsibility for careful monitoring of progress, assessment of emerging problems and taking action to help deal with these. Thus the program director's responsibilities might include formal monitoring of and feedback from the work environment (or other setting) by correspondence, email, or by visits to work settings where this is possible. Discussions with stakeholders is important such as with nurses' associations, government officials (including those who influence policy and planning decisions), and people in hospital or public health settings such as doctors, nurses and managers whose support is essential for successful outcomes of the different learning activities.

Program directors therefore need to work closely with the key stakeholders, as is relevant in different situations. Strategies will vary. Working together, it is possible to generate the enthusiasm and support that adds 'soul' to the leadership development experience in the work setting, for all concerned. The following example illustrates this enthusiasm from a key stakeholder, generated through the positive outcomes from participant team projects and in turn reinforcing to participants the importance of their development activities.

Health officials can contribute 'soul' to leadership development

'We [Trainer, President of the NNA and the ICN Consultant] met with the Minister of Health . . . everybody in the Ministry was sick with cold and flu symptoms, including the Minister, but he said he was excited to meet with us to discuss the success of the LFC™ program in his country. The Minister views the goals, objectives and outcomes of the program in line with his efforts to strengthen nurses' and midwives' leadership capacity in the nation.'[10] (Jamaica)

An increasing number of universities and other organizations in different countries are offering access to their programs to students from other countries, where the students remain in their home country and learn through distance learning, with teaching staff traveling to them for seminars and other aspects of course work. In these situations it is important that there is a close interface between university staff and local and national employers, to ensure that relevant factors from the work and political settings are integrated into program planning and implementation. A focus on the students only – the developing leaders – could be less effective in the longer term if the setting is not taken into account. This is a good example of where the process will be reflected in the outcome.

Some situations will dictate that a variety of personnel are included in discussions in the workplace. This depends on the nature of participant learning and activities, including team projects/syndicate work. It can have a number of benefits. Problems in the setting can be identified and acted on early. People in the setting feel involved and are more likely to cooperate with and give support to the developing leaders. They in turn feel supported and taken seriously, and better able to get maximum benefit from their learning activities.

Generating 'soul' in the setting

It was enlightening to see pride and a sense of helping to make a real difference, that cleaning staff exhibited when they were fully involved in projects to reduce hospital cross infection. And the enthusiasm and pleasure that volunteer workers demonstrated when contributing to projects in community public health settings.[11]

Taken together, these benefits can help pave the way for the emergence of 'soul' in leadership development. And it is soul shared with others that feeds back into the program (see below).

People contribute 'soul' to leadership development programs

The *doctors*, whose excitement over the results of a team project bring them to the final presentation of project outcomes, so they can support the team and lobby the program director and others to continue with this kind of leadership development program. For example: 'They have developed new strategies we hadn't thought of and the results are impressive . . . we will definitely be incorporating these strategies into our next (public health) programs.'[12] (Myanmar)

The *government health official*, who said 'It is unbelievable how they [the participants] have grown . . . they have developed assertive communication skills . . . they put in to practice what they have learned and interact well with all levels . . .'[13] (Seychelles)

(continued overleaf)

The *mentor*, who said 'I am the original mentor and for this team . . . I am proud, because all of my mentees hold the key for the future of nursing care in our nation.'[14] (Uganda)

The *nurses' association*, which was so pleased with a team project on mentoring that it published a small book on mentoring and made it widely available to nurses and hospital employers.[15] (Singapore)

The *Minister of Health*, who asked to meet with the country LFC™ team to hear what they had to say about what nurses could contribute to the planned health reforms. This demonstrated the value of forming strategic alliances with key stakeholders who really believe the [nursing] contribution can be important.[16] (St. Lucia)

The *public service*, in a small country in the Pacific which was impressed with the new performance appraisal system developed for nursing in the LFC™ country team project, and asked to adapt and adopt this for some other government departments and services.[17] (Kiribati)

Each of the above examples is from a different culture and a different part of the world: Latin America, the Caribbean, Asia, Africa and the Pacific. They illustrate not only the excitement, passion, inspiration and character (the 'soul') from leadership development in positive learning environments and settings, but that there *are* commonalities across cultures as we have asserted as a premise to this book.

The followers

Clearly the leader, the setting and the followers are overlapping and integrated components of leadership. And in leadership development the challenge is to develop the person's skills and confidence so they are better able to inspire, motivate and influence others including 'the followers'. How does a leadership development program do this?

A firm belief in action learning, or learning by doing, is asserted in this book. Not just as one segment or unit of a program, but as an integral part of all components. For example, formal lectures can be interspersed with action-learning activities that help develop leadership skills and behaviors. Other specific action-learning activities can be developed for a wide variety of topics such as working with the media, articulating the value of nursing to others, developing vision statements, project planning and implementation, self-assessment and peer review, analysis and critical feedback, role-play, making effective presentations, developing and implementing marketing plans, developing and implementing individual development plans, and many others. Such activities can motivate and influence others as they are being carried out. But they also develop a deeper capacity to transfer the skills and behaviors learned to other situations as a purposeful part of observable leadership behavior.

Developing skills and 'soul' through action learning

At workshops in the ICN LFC™ program, participants are often asked to articulate in front of the group the skills/attributes they have developed, and that other people have observed in them and commented on, in the months since the last workshop. Almost invariably the majority note:

- confidence (nearly always at the top of the list)
- motivation and self direction
- communication and listening skills
- priority setting
- teamwork and team building
- negotiation skills
- better focus, having a vision, setting targets
- more strategic and better able to plan ahead
- creative thinking and problem solving
- more objective self-assessment

Personal examples are given which are often quite moving, especially when they describe interaction with followers.[18]

Sometimes positive learning comes from potentially negative and very emotional experiences. Consider this example.

Action learning can produce powerful emotion

A role play was organized as a learning activity related to effective communication: learning to be clear and concise and very focused with busy and influential people. Two groups took part. One played the Minister of Health and his group (secretary/receptionist and various officials). The other played a small group of nurses who wanted to convey a message they felt passionately about. In the role play the 'Minister' was dismissive, disinterested, brusque and a bit belittling. The nurse spokesperson was upset, angry and tearful. The role play was terminated before it ended, for debriefing.

That evening, after the workshop session finished, a group of participants sat up into the night with some of the role players, to help support them and work through what had happened. The next day the 'nurse spokesperson' raised the situation during morning plenary. She explained that on reflection, the reason she had been so emotional was because she considered that was really the way nurses were often treated by officials – the 'Minister' had it right – and all her past frustrations and feelings of disempowerment just flowed over. This led into a broader discussion of self-awareness and how to manage one's emotions so as to achieve productive outcomes. Later in the program the 'nurse spokesperson' commented on the positive learning this incident had led to and how she was able to learn from this to manage difficult situations with others, including 'followers', successfully.[19]

For many people, a new sense of character and identity often emerges during a leadership development program and this is noticeable to others:[20]

> **Emergence of a new character and identity**
>
> 'The staff tell me that I am different . . . they don't usually explain this with words like "confidence" or "motivation" . . . but they seek me out more and ask my opinion on things.' (East, Central and Southern Africa)
>
> 'I am asked to do more in the organization.' (Caribbean)
>
> 'Other units have become really interested in what we (the project team) are doing . . . they want us to extend it to their wards . . . they are more willing to be involved than they were at the start.' (Bangladesh)
>
> 'People ask me what I do that makes me get different results from what they get.' (Mauritius)

This emergence of character and identity, together with more 'emotional' traits, are part of the 'soul' of leadership development. It is noticeable when the leader or developing leader attracts others, builds trust with his or her followers, inspires loyalty, encourages the development of others' potential, shows courage and a willingness to take appropriate risks, and is clearly committed to and motivated by explicit values and beliefs.

As noted in Chapter 3, current leadership literature gives more emphasis to human and personal qualities, and leadership is often viewed in a model stressing learning, listening, coaching, experimenting and networking with other leaders. These ideas focus on personal attributes such as confidence, ability to earn trust and respect, having good listening skills, giving encouragement, empowering others, leading by example, networking, taking risks and developing others as leaders. These were illustrated in the examples given above. They develop best through action-learning programs which can enhance human qualities and develop behavioral skills. Integrated with sound knowledge and understanding of leadership theory and practice, they enhance the leader's personal credibility in the eyes of the followers and other key stakeholders.

A ten-lesson framework for developing 'soul'

The research of Posner and Kouzes[21] has showed that leadership is an 'observable, learnable set of practices'.[22] This research suggests ten lessons for leadership developers. It is useful to test out the concept of 'soul' in leadership development by seeing how it relates to these ten lessons. In each of the lessons outlined below, quoted text from Posner and Kouzes enlarges on the meaning of each 'lesson'. The examples illustrating each lesson, with an emphasis on demonstrating 'soul' in developing leaders where this is apparent, are from ICN documents relating to their LFC™ program worldwide. The ten lessons are:

(1) Challenge provides the opportunity for greatness – in leading and learning to lead.
(2) Leadership is in the eye of the beholder.

(3) Credibility is the foundation of leadership.
(4) The ability to inspire a shared vision differentiates leaders from other credible sources.
(5) Without trust, you cannot lead.
(6) Shared values make a critical difference in the quality of life at home and at work.
(7) Leaders are role models for their constituents.
(8) Lasting change progresses one hop at a time.
(9) Leadership development is self-development.
(10) Leadership is not an affair of the head. It is an affair of the heart.

Lesson 1: Challenge provides the opportunity for greatness – in leading and learning to lead. 'When we think of leaders we often recall periods of turbulence, conflict, innovation and change . . . Cases [of personal bests] were about significant change . . . testimony to the power of challenging opportunities to provide for the expression of extraordinary leadership actions . . . exciting, exhilarating, rewarding and fun. Dull, routine, boring experiences did not provide the opportunity to excel or to learn . . . Only challenge presents the opportunity for greatness.'[23]

Examples: challenge helps leaders develop

Out of change, and some degree of resistance and conflict, come a number of examples of challenging opportunities promoting positive leadership development in the East, Central and Southern Africa region. The region has been undergoing significant change and health sector reform, moving from traditional bureaucratic systems to new systems promoting good resource management, and emphasis on performance and accountability. In Zambia, in a resource-strapped environment of continued high need and demand for health services, evidence of change in one developing leader was described by an observer as follows: 'The major change is how she relates to others in the field, interviewing, responding to people, being confident, identifying key persons in trying to promote change . . . patient care has changed. What she has gained is enthusiasm.'[24] And this developing leader related her view of leadership: 'You need to provide opportunity for nurses to express themselves, to help others. When you see initiative, you do not stifle it, you create pathways. You do not worry about status or your place in the hierarchy, it's not about feeling important, it's about seeing others come through your path – to be there to facilitate an environment where people can express themselves. As you treat people like this, they confide in you and begin to offer suggestions to you rather than offering deference to your position.'[25] (Zambia)

Lesson 2: Leadership is in the eye of the beholder. 'Constituents choose leaders. . . . The trappings of power and position may give someone the right to exercise authority, but we should never, ever mistake position and authority for leadership.'[26] Only when constituents believe that leaders are capable of meeting their hopes and aspirations can the leader mobilize their actions. 'And to be able to respond to the needs of others, leaders must first get to know their constituents

... leaders serve their constituents ... if [leaders] cannot respond to their aspirations, they will not follow'.[27]

Differences in perception of leadership outcomes

Differences in perception of leadership outcomes were revealed among stakeholders.[28] 'Positives' reported by NNAs included:

- determination to introduce changes in the workplace in managing health services
- introduction of LFC™ concepts into the curricula of nurses, showing a commitment to helping develop others
- a unique opportunity for developing young nurses with potential for leadership
- development of regional alliances and networks in and between a number of countries
- improvement or introduction of some sort of strategic planning.

However, some NNAs had different or opposing views, depending on the country situation:

- Some NNAs are less able to see the benefits.
- Nurses' education and further training have been insufficiently revised to promote leadership and locally influence health reform.

Similarly, differences in perception came through from health ministry officials and health leaders and managers:

- Improved health management skills.
- Better teamwork.
- Improved communication.
- Mobilization among nurse leaders has improved.
- Some changes (more often at the local level) have taken place in the domain of health policy and reform.

And:

- A few national projects developed in the program have not been completed or integrated.
- Little substantive advice from participants has been received by health managers.

There are many reasons for differences in perception of leaders and their actions. Sometimes they are resented by holders of positional power, who may feel threatened by their actions. Sometimes the student leaders may not have sufficiently involved key people, including followers, in their activities. They may not have tried to motivate others, or produced results important to others. Other times there may be unresolved difficulties in the setting. Whatever the reason(s), the leader needs to draw on those behavioral characteristics that are more reflective of 'soul', such as motivating self and others, communicating effectively especially in difficult situations, role-modeling passion and commitment in beliefs and actions. It is in these ways that people are brought together toward common goals and will work together in trying to achieve them.

Meeting the hopes and aspirations of all constituents is particularly evident when developing leaders motivate and influence others, as in the following examples.

Responding to the aspirations of others

'They want us to extend our project to other areas so more can benefit.'[29] (Myanmar, Bangladesh)

'Our team project changed the framework for quality nursing care.'[30] (Barbados)

More people want to do LFC™ . . . or some other form of leadership and management development.[31] (Countries globally)

Lesson 3: Credibility is the foundation of leadership. Research from respondents around the globe showed Posner and Kouzes that people 'want leaders who are honest, forward-looking, inspiring and competent' if they were to follow them. 'Credibility is the single most important asset a leader has.'[32]

Establishing credibility

'Not just to say words, but to be a doer of words . . .'[33] (Jamaica)

'It is very embarrassing for a [nurse] manager in a high position not to be able to utter a single word during discussions or meetings regarding health sector reforms and nursing issues . . . so training of this nature [leadership development] should be made available for all nurse managers.'[34] (East, Central and Southern Africa)

'She is next in line for promotion to the top job, but she never talks . . . in meetings she is silent and now people ask "Why do they send this person to important meetings when she never talks" . . .'[35]

Lesson 4: The ability to inspire a shared vision differentiates leaders from other credible sources. 'The domain of leaders is the future . . . Equally important, however, is the leader's capacity to enlist others to transform the vision into reality . . . to inspire others to share the dream.'[36]

Shared vision

'Together we made our dream – getting a nursing law for the country – come true.'[37] (Venezuela)

The NNA Barbados has a long-term vision to see leadership development (LFC™) implemented for nurses at all levels, starting in 2003 and going through to 2012. Many people are working toward this, and their inspiration to officials is seeing results in getting funding for their programs.[38] (Barbados)

Lesson 5: Without trust, you cannot lead. 'Leaders can't do it alone . . . it's a team effort . . . They must create a climate in which others feel powerful, efficacious and strong.' This climate then becomes a learning environment, rather than one that blames people for their mistakes. 'Leaders focus on fostering collaboration, strengthening others and building trust.'[39]

Developing trust

Most participants agree the 'action learning', especially the team project work, is a significant part of their leadership development. But it is not always easy. They encounter the highs and the lows of teamwork. 'Highs' occur when teams share responsibility evenly; are equally motivated to succeed; are willing to work with and involve others; seek and act on advice from others; implement successful strategies and see positive results; get good feedback from others; work with the strengths and also develop weaker areas in team members; accept responsibility as a team and do not blame other team members, or others outside the team, when they run into difficulties. When they learn to trust each other and work effectively as a team, and when the team produces outcomes that are perceived favorably, then others such as officials and colleagues in the work setting trust them too.

Participants also have 'lows'. But they usually learn from what at the time are negative experiences that sometimes generate high emotion. In one country, team-building with one team was severely hampered by total disagreement on the main aims of the project and interpersonal difficulties within the team. This impeded any progress until one part of the team was insistent on starting a second project as they felt they were unable to trust and work with the others. After a number of meetings with key people, responsibility was put on the full team to resolve their problems in an accountable and professional way. They finally decided to stay together, to work on improving their interpersonal difficulties and to keep one project but implement it as two subgroups that take account of geographical distances.[40] The final successful outcome was probably made easier by one person virtually withdrawing from the project in its latter stages. The basic problem was an interpersonal one founded in lack of trust and strong determination to assert one's individual will.

Lesson 6: Shared values make a critical difference in the quality of life at home and at work. 'What do I stand for? What do I believe in? Shared values, e.g. within an organization and with colleagues help everyone to pull in the same direction. There is less stress and people are able to do more. Shared values enable everyone to experience ownership in their organization.'[41]

Shared values

A number of LFC™ participants comment on values and leadership strategies they develop and then take into their home environment. Examples are fostering independence with accountability, sharing work to get more things accomplished and being more open in communication. Values are often made explicit at the time of developing vision statements and need to be agreed to by the group if the vision is to serve as a motivating force bringing nurses together and enabling full participation in action plans oriented to key strategic goals. Here are some examples of shared values made explicit and

(continued)

agreed by all, which have helped participant teams get successful outcomes from their team projects:

- Competency in nursing practice
- Accountability by nurses
- Open communication
- Quality care
- Customer satisfaction
- Education for nurses

And here are some examples of 'negative values' that were observable in less successful project teams:

- Communication not open
- Non-sharing of information
- Low participation of colleagues and key organizations
- Resistance to change in the setting
- 'Guarding' of positional authority
- Lack of support

Often the more negative values are oriented to self, i.e. people feel threatened personally, or consider their position or authority is threatened, or are jealous of the success of others, or are apathetic themselves therefore not willing to support others or new initiatives. Negative values also often derive from the organizational culture. However, positive values are usually oriented to patients, the community, the health care system and to colleagues, rather than being governed by personal attitudes and issues. They reflect the development of 'soul' – the emotion, identity and character of the leader – that enables the leader to focus on the positive values that others are able to share and utilize as they all move forward to achieving common goals.

Lesson 7: Leaders are role models for their constituents. 'People believe in actions more than in words.'[42] Leaders live their values and beliefs, not just talk about them. This gives credibility, trust and confidence.

Role models

'Leadership skills do not go unnoticed – others value and welcome feedback from nurse leaders.'[43] (Trinidad and Tobago)

'The mentor for the Samoa team is a role model for the whole Pacific – we can learn a lot from her . . . she is not just capable, she is wise . . . she is highly regarded by many others . . .'[44] (Pacific)

'As a result of my participation in an international nursing conference, I have had a number of invitations from other countries to share our experiences with health reform, and how we have promoted the contribution of nursing to change . . .'[45] (East, Central and Southern Africa)

'There is greater awareness now of the importance of nurse leaders . . .'[46] (Singapore)

Lesson 8: Lasting change progresses one hop at a time. Break big goals down into achievable parts. Assign responsibilities to each team member. 'Progress is always incremental . . . The key to lasting improvements is small wins.'[47]

Establishing lasting change

The strategic thinking and planning process used for the ICN LFC™ enables participants to achieve what they initially thought might not be possible. It allows groups to work toward their goals 'one hop at a time'. A sense of pleasure and enthusiasm grows as targets are realized, successes demonstrated, and encouragement and positive feedback received from key stakeholders. This in turn contributes to effective ongoing monitoring and to sustainability of project results.

A motivating statement quoted elsewhere in this book is the Chinese proverb that 'a thousand mile journey begins with the first step'. And, as Posner and Kouzes say, lasting change progresses one hop at a time.[48]

Lesson 9: Leadership development is self-development. 'Leadership development is essentially a process of self-development . . . Through self development comes the self confidence to lead . . . [this] comes from learning about ourselves – our skills, prejudices, talents and shortcomings . . . leadership can be learned . . . development is a continuous improvement process, not an event, a class, a book, or series of programs.'[49]

Self-development helps generate enthusiasm

- 'The best part was doing the individual development planning. I have taken many courses in leadership and management but I have never done any development of myself . . . just went to the courses and that was that. But now I have been able to develop a new step and start a new life as a leader.'[50] (Mauritius)
- 'I used to be shy . . . now I am no longer shy. I used to say nothing, now I am the teacher and love it. It has helped me be more strategic, more aware of the bigger picture and health systems . . . as a result of my development planning I am headed next to get my PhD in health policy.'[51] (Jamaica)

Thus leadership development should not finish when a program finishes, but continue though planned self-development including formal and informal education and career planning. Some of this continued development is in specific areas of knowledge and skill, and some of it is the continued development of specific leadership behaviors. When participants continue working with a mentor, and become engaged in mentoring others, the development of leadership behaviors is more likely to be enhanced.

Lesson 10: Leadership is not an affair of the head. It is an affair of the heart. 'Leadership is emotional . . . To lead others requires passionate commitment to a set of fundamental beliefs and principles, visions and dreams.'[52] And it requires commitment to and belief in the followers.

These words by Posner and Kouzes describe 'soul' as the term is used in this book.[53] Leadership development can be emotional too.

> **The 'soul' of leadership development**
>
> 'LFC™ changed my life . . . now I am a Trainer of the LFC™ and I get to see the joy of lives being changed every day . . . it is priceless.'[54] (Barbados)

This last quote in particular reflects, it is believed, a passionate commitment to, and belief in, the followers.

Exercises and discussion questions

(1) 'Soul' is used in this book to describe the emotion, identity and character of the leader that become important as they involve themselves in the leadership process. Convene a small discussion group of nurse leaders and consider this concept as it applies to you. Does your leadership exhibit 'soul'? If so, how does this impact on others?

(2) If you are a nurse educator, or a student in a leadership development program, consider if the development of 'soul' is given sufficient focus in the leadership development program.

(3) Following on from exercise 2, how might this be strengthened? Write down your ideas, using the 'ten-lesson framework' from this chapter. Make recommendations relevant to others for changes, justifying all arguments used.

References and notes

(1) Cammock, P. (2003) *The Dance of Leadership: The Call for Soul in 21st Century Leadership.* Auckland: Prentice Hall Pearson Education in New Zealand Ltd., p. 28.

(2) Posner, B.Z. and Kouzes, J.M. (1996) Ten lessons for leaders and leadership developers. *Journal of Leadership Studies*, 3 (3).

(3) Correspondence (2005) from ICN consultant following a monitoring visit for ICN LFC™ TOT Jamaica. ICN, unpublished.

(4) Report (2002) on monitoring visits by National Coordinator for ICN LFC™ TOT Bangladesh, 2002. ICN, unpublished.

(5) Project reports, observation, comment and feedback in the ICN LFC™ projects for Bangladesh. ICN, unpublished.

(6) Posner, B.Z. and Kouzes, J.M. (1996) Ten lessons for leaders and leadership developers. *Journal of Leadership Studies*, 3 (3).

(7) ICN notes, discussions and observation during ICN LFC™ program implementation.

(8) ICN (2002) (developed by James Buchan). *Impact and Sustainability of the Leadership For Change Project 1996–2000.* Geneva: ICN, pp. 5–33.

(9) Both examples (1997–2001) taken from documents, discussion and observation during and after ICN LFC™ implementation for these two small nations.

(10) Report (2005) on monitoring visit for ICN LFC™ TOT Jamaica. ICN, unpublished.
(11) ICN LFC™ program experience.
(12) Comment (2005) made at final presentations of team projects, ICN LFC™ TOT Myanmar, 2005.
(13) Quoted (2001) in the *Country Case Study for the Seychelles*, a component of the ICN LFC™ Evaluation Study 2000–2001. ICN, unpublished.
(14) Notes (2005) from discussion with key stakeholders during monitoring visit for ICN LFC™ TOT Uganda. ICN, unpublished.
(15) Verbal report (2001) to ICN from the Singapore Nurses Association.
(16) Verbal presentation (1997) during review of progress in ICN LFC™ Caribbean Phase 1. ICN, unpublished notes.
(17) Final presentation (1999) of team projects for ICN LFC™ Pacific. ICN, unpublished notes.
(18) Program documents and reports (1996–2005) ICN LFC™. ICN, unpublished.
(19) ICN consultant experience during implementation of ICN LFC™.
(20) The following examples are all taken from ICN LFC™ program documents and recorded discussion during workshops. ICN, unpublished.
(21) Posner, B.Z. and Kouzes, J.M. (1996) Ten lessons for leaders and leadership developers. *Journal of Leadership Studies*, 3 (3).
(22) *Ibid.*, p. 3.
(23) *Ibid.*, p. 4.
(24) Quoted (2001) in *Country Case Study for Zambia*, a component of the ICN LFC™ program evaluation 2000–2001. ICN, unpublished.
(25) *Ibid.*
(26) Posner, B.Z. and Kouzes, J.M. (1996) Ten lessons for leaders and leadership developers. *Journal of Leadership Studies*, 3 (3), 4–5.
(27) *Ibid.*, p. 5.
(28) Draft Report (2000) to ICN of *Questionnaires Analysis*, a component of the ICN LFC™ program evaluation 2000–2001. ICN, unpublished.
(29) Participant reports on team projects in hospital settings. ICN, unpublished.
(30) Participant comment (2005) during monitoring visit for ICN LFC™ TOT Barbados.
(31) Program documents, feedback and reports (1996–2005) for ICN LFC™, including data from the countries involved in the TOT (Training of Trainers) programs.
(32) Posner, B.Z. and Kouzes, J.M. (1996) Ten lessons for leaders and leadership developers. *Journal of Leadership Studies*, 3 (3), 5.
(33) Draft Report (2000) to ICN of *Questionnaires Analysis*, a component of the ICN LFC™ program evaluation 2000–2001. ICN, unpublished.
(34) East, Central and Southern Africa College of Nursing (ECSACON) (2003) *Report on Evaluation of the ECSA Leadership and Management Programme*. Arusha: ECSACON and the Commonwealth Regional Health Community Secretariat, p. 28.
(35) Comment to ICN consultant in a country that promotes on length of service, not merit.
(36) Posner, B.Z. and Kouzes, J.M. (1996) Ten lessons for leaders and leadership developers. *Journal of Leadership Studies*, 3 (3), 6.
(37) Correspondence (2005) to ICN from LFC™ graduate and now LFC™ Trainer for Venezuela.
(38) Report (2003) on monitoring visit for ICN TOT Barbados. ICN unpublished.
(39) Posner, B.Z. and Kouzes, J.M. (1996) Ten lessons for leaders and leadership developers. *Journal of Leadership Studies*, 3 (3), 7.
(40) Report (2003) to project stakeholders, ICN LFC™ in one country. ICN, unpublished.
(41) Posner, B.Z. and Kouzes, J.M. (1996) Ten lessons for leaders and leadership developers. *Journal of Leadership Studies*, 3 (3), 7.
(42) Posner, B.Z. and Kouzes, J.M. (1996) Ten lessons for leaders and leadership developers. *Journal of Leadership Studies*, 3 (3), 8.

(43) Participant comment in *Nursing in the Caribbean, a Story of Leadership* (2002) Publication prepared by Wendy Kitson-Piggott, ICN Regional Project Leader for the Caribbean team. ICN LFC™ publication.

(44) Participants' comments, expressed during the Pacific ICN LFC™ commencing 1998 and involving five Pacific countries. This mentor talked frankly and openly with all Pacific participants about her nursing leadership journey.

(45) Participant comment in written report on progress with ECSACON/ICN LFC™. ICN, unpublished.

(46) Comment (2000) by non-participant beneficiary, in Draft Report to ICN of *Questionnaires Analysis*, a component of the ICN LFC™ program evaluation 2000–2001. ICN, unpublished.

(47) Posner, B.Z. and Kouzes, J.M. (1996) Ten lessons for leaders and leadership developers. *Journal of Leadership Studies*, 3 (3), 8.

(48) Posner, B.Z. and Kouzes, J.M. (1996) Ten lessons for leaders and leadership developers. *Journal of Leadership Studies*, 3 (3), 8.

(49) *Ibid.*, p. 9.

(50) ICN LFC™ documentation. ICN, unpublished.

(51) *Ibid.*

(52) Posner, B.Z. and Kouzes, J.M. (1996) Ten lessons for leaders and leadership developers. *Journal of Leadership Studies*, 3 (3), 9.

(53) The notion of 'soul' is described in Chapter 2 as the emotion, identity and character of the leader, from Cammock, P. (2003) *The Dance of Leadership: The Call for Soul in 21st Century Leadership.* Auckland: Prentice Hall Pearson Education in New Zealand Ltd., p. 28.

(54) Trainer comment (2003) to ICN consultant during monitoring visit for ICN LFC™ TOT Barbados.

Chapter 7
Leadership in practice: outcomes for the person

How are the results of leadership and leadership development measured? Indeed, can they be measured or is it more like an observable set of frequently recurring 'best practices'? Is it to be seen in individual development, or in the ability to 'create more leaders'? Is it in the effectiveness of new systems and processes? Or in the outcomes of specific projects? What makes a leader effective? Most probably it is a bit of all of these.

Leadership development programs are marketed by their products. The primary product is the person being developed as a leader. Secondary products are the outcomes of that person's leadership activities. Both contribute to the reputation and image of the organization providing the leadership development program. This helps gain stakeholder support, which is necessary for further programs and any funding proposals to support these.

This chapter uses the 'person' component of the now familiar framework of person, setting and followers, using primarily examples from the International Council of Nurses Leadership for Change™ (ICN LFC™) experience. It starts with initial selection into a leadership development program and then the individual development outcomes that can be expected. The 'setting' and the 'followers' are addressed in Chapter 8. The setting (environment of leadership) will look at how leaders can influence policy and changes in organizations and health systems (and indeed be influenced by them) and then outcomes for the followers are considered – those who are influenced by the leadership development process of their colleagues, during and after formal programs. Evidence of 'soul' is illustrated in different examples in both Chapters 7 and 8.

Selection influences results

Initial selection of people into a program can help determine results. Some leadership development programs allow people to self-select for entry, i.e. if they wish to do the program and places are available then they can enter. Other programs have firm criteria for selection, including academic and/or previous experience. Sometimes there are selection criteria but these are influenced by political or economic pressures. Reasons for the different approaches, or some modification of these, are varied. They often include:

- revenue to the organization offering the program
- policy and criteria of the primary funder(s)
- status: the desire that only people of a certain caliber graduate
- need: the desire to spread the opportunity for development broadly, based on health service needs; or the desire to target specific groups.

Some criteria focus on both the person and the setting. And if we look closely at the criteria on some application forms, we might see some hint of a search for 'soul' in questions relating to, for example, vision, commitment, or motivation. Perhaps selection criteria should look more actively for the potential for 'soul', such as passion, excitement, motivation and the ability to motivate others, at the selection stage. In some settings, requirements for previous academic qualifications have less relevance such as in countries where opportunity and access to obtaining qualifications are more limited. Some providers of programs recognize this by formalizing criteria which will give 'recognition of prior learning'.

Gaining language skills

Language is often a challenge in leadership development in a cross-cultural context. Increasingly, the English language is becoming the language of professional communication in nursing and health care (as in other fields). Language determines access to resource material available through the internet as well as many libraries. It facilitates communication, for example by email. It enables better communication across a variety of cultures. Indeed, the English language is increasingly the language of communication between two cultures where English is the second language of both, not the first. Program providers therefore need to take language into account in initial selection of participants. Some provide facilities for selected participants to learn English as a second language prior to course commencement, or provide interpretation in the formal education setting. Some provide for translation of resource materials and on-site interpretation. Others have a requirement that the national coordinator for an in-country program with external providers, has a reasonable command of English, if this is the main language of communication with the external provider.

Outcomes from mentoring and individual development planning

Working with a mentor is an essential component of leadership development. There should be benefits for both the mentor and the mentee. In Chapter 5 mentoring was discussed in the context of designing a successful program. It was noted that a successful mentor–mentee relationship depends on:

- the selection and skills of the mentor
- the motivation and commitment of both parties
- investment of time
- commitment
- clarity and mutual understanding of the role
- the right 'chemistry' between mentor and mentee.

Not all mentor–mentee relationships have positive results. In general, they are probably more successful when the mentee selects their mentor themselves, than when the mentor self-selects or is 'appointed' by others. Here are some comments by mentors in three different regions about good outcomes they consider they have contributed to.[1]

Mentor contributions to participant outcomes

'The participants have made a breakthrough in their development . . . most importantly, they developed self confidence . . . there has been increased motivation and attitudinal changes . . .' (Caribbean)

'It helped increase their knowledge . . . there is better group work and team building . . . it helped strengthen and clarify the aptitudes of a leader.' (Latin America)

'It gave moral support and guidance, though there is still room for improvement in all areas . . . it has provided for capacity building on a continuous basis at minimal cost . . . it contributes to team cohesiveness and to project success . . . it creates confidence . . . (East, Central and Southern Africa)

Mentees themselves have of course much to do with positive outcomes, especially if they are prepared to put the time and effort into the relationship. Sometimes they have to go that bit further to overcome perceived obstacles.

Mentoring obstacles

'The mentor was hard to get hold of . . . always busy . . . couldn't give the time . . .'[2]

Where a strong and mutually beneficial mentor–mentee relationship develops, there should be positive outcomes for both. The *mentor* is constantly reviewing trends and issues in the external environment; reviewing and expanding knowledge; keeping up with the literature so as to be able to refer relevant articles and books to the mentee; and continuing to develop skills in coaching, debating, challenging and supporting. The *mentee* is exposing ideas and plans to review and debate; gaining information; acquiring skills; and learning how to become a mentor to others.

How mentoring helps development outcomes

'My mentor kept me focused on my objectives in order to meet the [longer term] goal . . . and other nurses I have mentored have become very active and proactive.'[3] (Uganda)

Individual development planning is another important component of an effective leadership development program. Development plans can take a variety of formats, but usually entail the participant/student reviewing the factors in themselves or their setting that might help or hinder their development, then setting two or three specific goals each year, with planned activities and clear timelines, to meet their individual development needs. The outcomes might be more measurable, as in acquiring computer skills, or much more difficult to achieve and demonstrate to others, such as developing political skills, or becoming more motivated and motivating others. Here are some examples of outcomes achieved in the course of a leadership development program, where students focused on areas of development that were specific to their own needs.

> **Examples of outcomes from individual development planning**
>
> - Obtain further academic qualifications
> - Prepare oneself to become chief nurse
> - Self-development and self-evaluation
> - Improved focus, motivation, will power
> - Improved communication, political and negotiation skills
> - Ability to envision
> - Progress with English language skills
> - Financial management skills
> - Extended networks
> - Computer skills
> - Increased self-confidence
> - Learned to become a good mentor

Other outcomes in individual development

In Chapter 3 a number of characteristics, or 'traits' of leadership, that most would acknowledge as key attributes of an effective leader were identified. However, it was cautioned against defining leadership only in these terms. A theoretical approach that takes account of the leader, the setting and the followers was subscribed to. This integrated approach has been used as a basic framework in this book. Later, in Chapter 8, possible results, or outcomes, in terms of the setting and the followers will be explored. But first, the leader.

Key attributes of leadership, although of course not necessarily all, were outlined in Chapter 3. These are summarized in Box 7.1.

Most of the above characteristics should show some development early in a leadership program. The evidence can be obtained through some or all of the following, depending on the nature of the program.

- observation in the learning environment (formal education plus work or professional setting)
- reports of progress from/discussion with colleagues
- progress with individual development and career planning
- reports of progress with and from mentors

- self-assessment
- peer review
- reports of promotion or involvement in other work or professional committees and activities
- progress with special projects and other structured learning and development activities.

Box 7.1   Some key attributes of leadership

- The ability to envision a desired future and to think strategically
- External awareness
- Influence
- Self-motivation
- The ability to motivate, inspire and influence others
- Confidence in self, and the ability to inspire confidence in others
- Credibility and trust
- Political skill
- Review, change and renewal – the ability to continually challenge and develop self, review directions and strategies, and foster the development of others
- Teamwork, partnerships and collaboration
- Communication skills

In some ways, results in individual development are usually easier and quicker to see than results in the setting and in the followers. But it depends on the degree of motivation, the nature and extent of action learning and related activities and the extent to which factors in the environment (or setting) are conducive to change. Sometimes these factors overcome other potential barriers, such as perceived status in a hierarchical system. However, even given the most encouraging environment, there are always some individuals who are just not able to make the most of the learning opportunities provided. Following are some examples of outcomes beginning to emerge for the person (as opposed to setting and followers) early on in a leadership development program.

Early outcomes for individuals

After six months, most participants were taking formal lessons in English. Fifteen participants had taken formal classes in computer skills and internet and email use. They had negotiated with their supervisors for new computers and printers in their work settings. Ten of 27 participants had achieved approval to attend school for a higher nursing degree.[4] (Mongolia)

In the East, Central and Southern Africa (ECSA) program, the most important learning after the first workshop was identified as:

- Negotiation skills
- Strategic thinking and planning
- Developing a vision and being visionary

(continued)

Participants were also asked to record, after the first workshop, the most significant learning for them personally. Here is what some of them said:

- 'I have had to re-look at myself [in the changing environment of health care in her country], and have found I have weaknesses that need to be addressed – I shall be able to strengthen these areas.'
- 'I am better able to think on my feet.'
- 'It has enabled me to think and sort my ideas in a more organized way, thereby bringing better results.'
- 'To manage change is not easy; one has to be prepared for it and have courage and perseverance.' (East, Central and Southern Africa)

In the United Arab Emirates, participants noted growth in the following areas after six months:

- Confidence, motivation and commitment
- Vision and strategic planning
- Communication
- Time management
- Negotiation
- Cooperation and teamwork.[5] (United Arab Emirates)

As leadership development programs progress, students are exposed to increasing opportunities for action learning, both in the 'safe' environment of the workshops or other education setting and in the real – and often difficult – environment of their work settings. Leadership attributes continue to develop, practiced in the educational environment and nurtured by structured learning activities in their own professional and employment settings.

Effort produces better outcomes

'Those individuals who participated most frequently and intensively in the projects, experienced the greatest changes in their motivation, capacity and performance.'[6]

Certain outcomes for individuals should be well established by the end of a program. The following examples represent the most significant areas of individual development across quite different cultures, organizations and country situations.[7]

Outcomes at the end of a program

- Confidence
- Communication skills
- Vision and strategic thinking
- Influence and negotiation
- Developing and extending networks and alliances, coordinating and working more effectively with officials and other stakeholders and getting support and cooperation

(continued overleaf)

- Team building and working effectively in teams
- Project planning, implementation and management skills, including writing grant proposals, report writing and budget planning and management
- Motivation
- External awareness
- Improved use of technology

Other outcomes reported by different people, that are less common but nevertheless important include:

- Speaking up in meetings and public forums
- More energized
- Better able to compromise
- Better able to deal with uncertainty
- Able to articulate policy issues during health reform
- Having a positive 'can do' attitude
- Having a better orientation to and focus on customers/clients
- Greater decisiveness
- Creative and more analytical thinking
- Better problem solving and decision-making
- Better time management
- Learning to achieve results within constraints
- Self direction
- Better interpersonal relationships
- More capacity for tolerance and control of emotions.

Outcomes in individual development should become obvious to colleagues and others, not just 'felt' by the person themselves. This is reflected in the following examples.

Participant outcomes described by others

'It has been a fascinating experience to observe the growth in participants over the past 2–4 years as they have worked through the action-learning process. In the main, they have become far more resourceful, more patient, willing and able to negotiate at the highest decision-making levels, and better able to organise their time and respond to the many demands that leaders face on a daily basis. They have become more accepting of and more responsive to the responsibility they hold for the development of their peers. They have begun to seriously consider taking the risks they need to if they are to achieve their goals. Several of them have demonstrated this in no uncertain manner, leaving the comfort of "safe" jobs for more risky but challenging and exciting endeavours.'[8] (Caribbean region)

A number of important areas of individual growth were observed in participants in the Latin America region. These included accepting responsibility for development of self and other leaders, working more collaboratively and in strategic alliances, and being more prepared to take on leadership roles in management, at universities and

(*continued*)

in policy. Some reported professional growth leading to job promotions, and more involvement in policy at national and international level. Most agreed on increased self-direction, decision-making skills, improved teamwork, a clearer understanding of the effects of political and other factors on health; and a strengthened capacity in communication (oral and written). There were developments in planning and organizing, working with key stakeholders; networking; oral and written presentations; using technology; mentoring other nurses; negotiation skills; and development of strategies with national nurses' associations (NNAs) that enabled greater thinking and knowledge about health reform.[9] (Latin America region)

Possibly the most universally reported area of development has been the growth of confidence in self. You will recall from Chapter 3 that Kanter[10] drew a distinction between two different aspects of confidence: the self-confidence of the leader and the broad sense of whether people have confidence in their leader. But she also believes that although many leaders have self-confidence, this is not the real secret of leadership. Rather, the more essential ingredient is whether they (the leaders) have confidence in other people and therefore can create the conditions in which the people they lead can get the work done. Having confidence in other people underpins at least some of the other 'themes' identified above: first, developing and extending networks and alliances, coordinating and working more effectively with officials and other stakeholders, and getting support and cooperation; and second, team-building and working effectively in teams.

Confidence is a concept that can be expressed differently in different cultures. In some parts of Africa, for example, not being confident can be described as 'being shy'.

> **What the words really mean: the example of confidence**
>
> 'I was shy, so shy . . . now I am a leader . . . I am ready for the challenge.' (East, Central and Southern Africa)
>
> 'We are no longer the shy girls of [our country] . . . rather, we are leaders.'[11] (East, Central and Southern Africa)
>
> 'I realized that before I trained, I was rather shy, but now I am more vocal and confident.'[12] (East, Central and Southern Africa)

'Being shy' was also described as part of the culture in Singapore. The following example illustrates growing confidence in a group of participants in a leadership development program.

> 'This event . . . was a grand time with 27 nations represented and more than 75 nurses. Around 50 plus Singapore nurses were invited. The participants had a great time practicing their communication and networking skills, and I had a great time watching them go around and meet and greet every participant at the reception. It was impressive to watch . . . Prior to their participation in the program, these participants were described as very shy.'[13] (Singapore)

Confidence can also underlie other leadership skills, such as problem solving.

'Their perception of problems and difficulties changed as they gained skill, confidence and motivation in problem solving. What would have been considered a problem earlier, was viewed differently later in the program'.[14] (Bangladesh)

The impact of continuing effective leadership behavior

Regardless of a person's development and progress during a leadership development program, it is what happens after this that really counts. Development of leadership attributes that are 'turned off' at program's end, or only given lip service to, is a failed development opportunity. Already it has been seen how the setting is an important component of leadership and leadership development. The role of the setting in helping sustain individual development will be discussed in Chapter 9 on sustainability of outcomes. However, the person cannot rely solely on the setting, or make excuses that to exercise leadership in their setting, the setting must be different. For surely part of the role of the leader is to help initiate and bring about change in settings that desperately need it. It may be tough, but embarking on the leadership journey means committing oneself to these challenges.

Effective leadership behavior means having an impact on setting and followers. It is initiating needed changes and following through to the achievement of clear results and outcomes. For many, it is being active and successful in influencing policy, and in motivating and influencing others to achieve common goals. It is looking ahead and planning strategically to meet longer-term goals. It is being creative in proposing solutions and strategies rather than being bound by the status quo. It is communicating, being both confident and credible, working with others to achieve results, and encouraging the formation of strategic partnerships and alliances.

Credibility and working with others to achieve results[15]

'When I went with N. to the Ministry of Health, he helped to increase the salaries of not just the nurses but of other professionals, such as laboratory, social workers and others, and also increased allowances for medical care, housing and uniforms stipends. I was impressed with his style of negotiation and his patience; he was professional and well prepared, and clear on what they would negotiate vs. what they would not. But, most importantly, I got to see the true expressions of gratitude and warmth towards him from those representing the other health professionals. They were holding on to his every word and were in agreement with his negotiating arguments. He is making changes not just for the nurses but for all the health professionals and ultimately for the people in the nation.'

It may be a good idea at this stage for readers to go back and review Chapters 3 and 4 which are about leadership – the person, the setting and the followers. This will help to create a mental picture of what leadership is about, so effective leadership behaviors seen in self and in others can be reviewed.

Effective leadership behaviors that continue into the longer term should have an impact on the setting and on the followers. Consider the following examples.

The impact individuals can have on organizations

Individuals can contribute to:[16]

- The development of a strategic management culture
- Better management of change
- New ways of thinking how to handle health reform challenges
- Higher motivation of management, for change and of staff to the organization
- More positive nurse attitudes towards patients
- Less complaints of health care provided
- A lot of interest in self-development
- Expanded teamwork.

Individuals gained new knowledge and skill and also:[17]

- 'Changed' some perceptions of nursing as a profession
- Made participants more confident, resourceful and ready to talk to superiors and the public
- Empowered some NNAs, helping them become more structured and strategic in addressing professional and membership issues
- Strengthened organizational capacity, for example the ability to deal with changes related to national health reform.

The development of effective nurse leaders can, in countries where the status of women and of nursing in society is low, help change perceptions of nursing as a profession. Usually this change comes about at an organizational level, where the impact of leadership behaviors may be more obvious. But changes can be observed at a national level also. What makes the difference is often the demonstrable differences the nurse leaders make through their project work and results during a program, and their continued leadership behavior and its results after programs end. But additionally, working with an expanded group of key stakeholders, and demonstrating leadership skills at an individual level as well as providing evidence through the changes these skills help bring about, nurses, doctors, health officials, the public and others become convinced that nursing does have much of value to offer. This is reflected in the following comments.

Helping to change perceptions on the value of nursing

'The achievement of social recognition for nursing is a medium range result, nevertheless, it is gratifying to see the recognition for country participants, mainly for one of them who is respected like an expert in the area of management and leadership for change™.'[18] (Latin America)

'The image of nursing has improved with Doctors, managers and patients.'[19] (Bangladesh)

This value is often translated into concrete action by involving nurses in multidisciplinary committees and related activities and promoting nurses to other positions because of the leadership and management skills they demonstrate. Some individual nurses also seek greater involvement in health policy and planning, and in taking on a variety of leadership roles in professional and community affairs. Following are some examples of positive outcomes that have impact, or the strong potential for impact because of the leadership roles occupied and the leadership behaviors demonstrated to others.

Impact of leadership development

(a) *Assuming leadership roles and positions*

'The people from this program are growing personally and professionally in dynamic and exciting ways. Several . . . are in line for, or have achieved, promotion to various leadership positions in government and as matrons of local hospital systems; one has been promoted to be an Assistant Director for the Drug and Crime Prevention program for the nation, others are eager to pursue leadership positions in their National Nurses' Association, such as President and Vice President. One is the new President of their regional nursing organization.'[20] (Caribbean and Latin America)

(b) *Officials promise funding for future programs*

'The Permanent Secretary was impressed with the excellent individual development that she had seen . . . as a result of this she announced that the government would be paying for future programs, and that acting positions for nurse leaders in the Ministry of Health (CNO and Deputy CNO) would be put on permanent status. The Permanent secretary said "I see the changes, and that nurses are giving us the products we need to change policies in our health system".'[21] (Mauritius)

(c) *Involvement in the training and education of others*

'All the current participants plan to actively assist the certified trainers with future programs, in the roles of mentors and team project advisors. They are now more confident in their skills in negotiation, strategic thinking and planning, political astuteness and communication, and say their leadership development has made the difference in the way they live and work as nurse leaders and managers.'[22] (Barbados)

Earlier in this section it was asserted that the person (the leader) cannot rely solely on the setting, or make excuses that to effectively exercise leadership their setting must be change and be different. Part of the role of the leader is to help initiate and bring about change in settings that desperately need it . . . and embarking on the leadership journey means committing oneself to these challenges.

The following case study, from Nicaragua, demonstrates how leaders can respond positively to difficult challenges in their environment, to bring about change. In this case study the essence was commitment, perseverance and the ability to motivate others to have an impact on nursing and health services through their actions.

Commitment and perseverance: case study from Nicaragua[23]

This country has been characterised by political instability, with many changes in government officials. This is reflected in the health system, which is characterised by many changes in leadership and again little stability. When this country planned to implement Trainer-led LFC™ (TOT), there was only one certified Trainer, and an ambitious proposal to implement a program for sixty people. The Provider Organization was the [main funder]. The Trainer was their head co-ordinator for the entire country, and therefore well positioned to facilitate the LFC™ through the foundation, and to get funding support. The foundation paid for LFC™ because the nurse participants also implement foundation strategies through the ministry of health. Sixty of one hundred and twenty nurses employed by the MOH in this region were selected to do the initial Trainer-led LFC™ program, funded by the [main funder] up to 2005. This helped to get it established in the country and paved the way for program continuation if other stakeholders could be convinced of its benefits.

However, there were some difficulties the Trainer had to overcome. One major issue was in communications with a key stakeholder because of their different political views. In this case, the Trainer and the stakeholder 'agreed to disagree' on issues relevant to both of their political parties, and they are working together to ensure the success of the LFC™ initiative. This took work on both sides to reach this agreement, and a need to keep focused on the outcomes desired (support for continuing the LFC™ initiative in the country) rather than on possible political impediments. None-the-less, political issues do impact on health services.

Another key stakeholder and potential funder for further programs was not interested in the LFC™ because he considered it was too long and it would be difficult to make a real difference. His view was that a program on the web using distance-learning technologies to reach a larger audience would be more appropriate, and that nurses should be studying public health and epidemiology rather than leadership as this was what the real priorities for the country were based on. He was unable to assist with further funding and said that there were greater needs for nursing in the country. This person later left the post, which was vacant for some time, making it difficult for continuity of ideas and action. However the position was later filled, and funding for LFC™ made available.

On the plus side was the key support of the Assistant Minister of Health, who was impressed with the LFC™ initiative and the participants' team projects, and requested to meet with the Trainer again to strategize on a plan to implement the LFC™ TOT initiative throughout Nicaragua.

A key Medical Director and Chief Nursing Officer also supported the program and were pleased with the emerging outcomes for participants as individuals, and for their team projects.

So at the time when the initial program was finishing and further programs needed funding support, the strengths in the situation could be summarized as:

- a strong Trainer, with the respect of her peers
- Trainer on the Executive Board of the NNA
- support of the NNA (although no funding available from this source)

(*continued overleaf*)

- Trainer active in the region of the initial program as a former politician and well-known public health nurse
- strong partnership between the [main funder] and the regional Ministry of Health
- a good rapport between the Trainer and the Assistant Minister of Health, with the potential to expand the LFC™ TOT initiative in Nicaragua
- initiative demonstrated by participants in obtaining funding support for team projects
- enthusiasm and commitment of participants
- positive outcomes demonstrated in the initial Trainer-led LFC™ team projects.

Those participant projects able to get funding and that were supported by a variety of key stakeholders were:

- training community leaders in leadership and strengthening community organization
- establishing clubs in the community for elderly people with chronic depression
- equipping a maternity ward
- forming a group of breast feeding donor mothers to improve a milk bank
- quality management in one municipality
- establishing a hostel for pregnant women from inaccessible areas in the region who are in the initial stages of labour and in need of care in the adult emergency ward of the regional Hospital
- educating, and establishing a network for, adolescents on issues relating to reproductive risk factors, to reduce the number of adolescent pregnancies
- promotion of the proper use of foods to improve the nutritional state of children under five
- training third year students at a school of nursing in innovative methodologies for managing change in adolescent pregnancy prevention.

On the other hand, weaknesses were identified as:

- no firm funding received for program continuity
- the [main funder] leaving the country.

Both these were later remedied.

In this situation the Trainer has demonstrated tenacity, commitment and perseverance. She has implemented a program for sixty participants virtually single-handed, but with excellent support from mentors. She had tried to deal with negative influences in the environment, or setting. She mobilized some funding and equipped program participants with skills to also seek funding for team projects. She has promoted and overseen team projects linked to important health priority areas for the nation. At the same time, although she was given some time off from her job for the LFC™ implementation, she has still fulfilled some responsibilities for her job and has continued as an Executive Board member for the NNA. The key to continued success will rest with continuity of LFC™ in the country and training of further Trainers.

The following set of examples from Venezuela show how leadership skills can be used strategically and in an innovative way to benefit others.

Being strategic: examples from Venezuela[24]

A strategic initiative relates to the need to generate funding for the ongoing implementation of leadership development programs. A Foundation for Leadership was started, to take donations from hospitals and companies to sponsor the LFC™ program. It helps them pay for the books and the venue, nursing leadership symposia and other related events.

A further initiative which is strategic in enhancing the image and value of nursing in the society is the creation of the national award for added value in nursing in the areas of: Care, Teaching and Research. The competition is held every year, with the participation of all nurses who have added value to nursing. This award has enabled the following:

- improved health and nursing services
- created and improved continuing education programs
- increased the amount of research in health and nursing
- improved sharing of professional and scientific information for nursing professionals in Venezuela.

The award is granted by the Federation of Nursing Colleges of Venezuela and the Centre of Research Information and Documentation in Venezuela. This is a good example of a strategic alliance.

Another good example of being strategic is in promoting health and through this, enhancing the image and visibility of nursing. Leaders in the Trainer-led LFC™ program took part in a 'demonstration' in the streets of a town where they discussed the health risks of tobacco dependence. In another town, a team worked together with the NGO 'Amigos Solidarios' on the Jornada de Salud ('day of health'), providing their professional services free of charge for the community, and leading educational discussions on the prevention of teenage pregnancies, domestic violence and drug abuse.

Finally, being strategic can also mean demonstrating to funders the benefits to them from good leadership development outcomes, thereby gaining additional funding for further programs.

Developing self through developing others

Individual development continues when former students/participants in leadership development programs are involved in developing others. This is illustrated in the following two brief case studies.

Case study: developing self through developing others

In 1996, two separate ICN LFC™ programs commenced with five countries for the Caribbean and five countries in Latin America. Both were funded by the W.K. Kellogg Foundation. On completion of these programs ICN was invited by the funder to submit a further proposal for a Phase 2 program, involving more countries and using some of the Phase 1 participants as coaches and mentors.

(continued overleaf)

Three further Caribbean countries were involved. All remaining Latin American countries were invited; all but two accepted. There were two participants from the new Latin America countries, one from each of the three new Caribbean countries, and one from each of the ten Caribbean and Latin America countries in Phase 1. It was agreed to structure the new Phase 2 as one combined program, with four regional teams. Meetings and workshops of the full group were conducted through simultaneous translation and by use of one-to-one interpretation, or by use of own language combined with gestures and other nonverbal communication.

Four regional teams were formed, each with a contracted part-time regional project leader who was a person from the region with experience and skills in project management. The role of the project leader was mainly to coordinate the team at regional level, to facilitate the planning and implementation of regional team projects, and to promote ongoing development through regional activities. The ten participants who had been through Phase 1 worked closely with the regional project leader in various roles, including acting as 'coach' to new participants. This was planned to be part of the continuing development of the ten original Phase 1 participants. It involved working with the new Phase 2 participants to coach, guide and assist them with their individual leadership planning and development.

In addition to the continued development of the ten Phase 1 participants through this activity, the remaining Phase 1 participants were connected to Phase 2 through their continuing country projects. Some attended regional meetings. Thus the majority of the original 30 participants in the Caribbean and Latin America had opportunities for ongoing development and extended networks.

The reports of the four regional project leaders, and the growth and development of the new Phase 2 participants, attested to the leadership qualities of the Phase 1 participants who had a key role (for example, as 'coaches') in Phase 2. Thus, through contributing to the development of others, one continues to develop self.[25]

Case study: Training of Trainers (TOT)

This provides a further opportunity for individuals to continue to develop self through developing others. Implemented in 2002, it was based on lessons learned and teaching/learning resources developed over the initial years of the ICN LFC™. Opportunities were provided for some of the earlier countries to participate in TOT, and now it is offered routinely as an extension of all LFC™ programs. A group of LFC™ participants is selected by discussion between ICN and country stakeholders, and with participants themselves, and they complete a TOT workshop run by ICN. They then become licensed by ICN as TOT-certified LFC™ trainers. These trainers implement the next generation program(s). They are supported by a provider organization. The program, trainer and provider organization all form part of an ICN credentialing process, and are monitored on an annual basis. In this way the trainers have a unique opportunity to continue their own development by developing others and to work within a structured process with set standards against which performance can be assessed.

(continued)

Trainers need not be teachers in their professional capacity. Rather, they need to role-model leadership behaviors, and be able to impart knowledge and motivate, stimulate and encourage the next generation of leaders. They must be credible to their peers and well supported by colleagues and employing authorities. Trainers are sometimes uncertain and a bit lacking in self-confidence when selected for this role, but almost without exception they grow in confidence and competence as programs are implemented and the new participants demonstrate their growth and development as leaders.

To support the trainers, and provide further opportunity for their own ongoing development, the other participants from the first program are encouraged – indeed expected – to take some role in the new program. This may be as mentors, or in supporting project and other activities, or coaching on individual development plans.

In both of the case study examples above, the observable development outcomes for those involved in developing others are:

- mentoring, coaching and teaching skills
- further development of confidence
- sustained commitment and motivation
- more complete understanding of some knowledge areas such as health reform, quality improvement, data collection and analysis, financial management
- firmer desire to lead and to make a difference.

These development outcomes can still be achieved despite any difficulties that might exist in the setting, such as more limited stakeholder support.

In this chapter we have focused on outcomes of leadership development for the person – the individual who is the leader, or learning to be a leader. Outcomes for the setting and the followers will be discussed next, in Chapter 8.

Exercises and discussion questions

(1) You are probably a leader, or a person being developed as a leader. Write down the leadership attributes that *you* consider have developed further in you. Now write down those attributes that *others have told you* they consider to have been developed further in you. Identify any key differences and discuss these with your mentor.

(2) A person's leadership activities also produces outcomes, or results. Discuss with a group of 'followers', outcomes they have *observed* as a result of your leadership activities.

(3) An integral part of effective leadership is confidence:
  - confidence in self;
  - confidence in others;
  - others having confidence in the leader.

(4) Reflect on your own leadership practice and identify specific examples for each of the three types of confidence outlined above. What outcomes were there, for each of the examples?

(5) Continuing development of self usually takes place when a leader is involved in some way in the development of others. How do you contribute to the development of others? Write this down, then discuss it with those whose development you contribute to.

(6) In *your* view, what have you gained? In *their* view, what have they gained?

References and notes

(1) The comments from different regions are taken from respondent questionnaires used in the ICN LFC™ evaluation study, 2000–01. The region rather than the specific country has been given to uphold the confidentiality of the individual respondents to the questionnaires.

(2) These were frequently recurring comments from ICN LFC™ participants. But mentees have a responsibility to do their utmost to make the relationship work, or to end the relationship and find another mentor, or to share the role with more than one mentor.

(3) Participant report on progress during the ECSACON/ICN LFC™, 1998–2001.

(4) Reports (2004 and 2005) after second and third workshops for ICN LFC™ Mongolia. Unpublished.

(5) Report (2002) after the second workshop for ICN LFC™ UAE. Unpublished.

(6) East, Central and Southern Africa College of Nursing (ECSACON) (2003) *Report on Evaluation of the ECSA Leadership and Management Programme*. Arusha: ECSACON and the Commonwealth Regional Health Community Secretariat, p. iv.

(7) Data are from the ICN LFC™ and have been drawn from documentation relating to self-assessment, peer review, evaluation and formal observation and feedback from the groups; self-reporting of what others say; discussion and observation with program coordinators and other stakeholders; review of progress with team projects, mentoring and individual development plans; performance in the various learning activities; and monitoring visits by national coordinators.

(8) Final Report (2001) by Regional Team Leader for the Caribbean region in the ICN LFC™ Phase 2 program for the Caribbean and Latin America. ICN, unpublished.

(9) Final Report (2001) by Regional Team Leaders for three Latin America regions in the ICN LFC™ Phase 2 program for the Caribbean and Latin America. ICN, unpublished.

(10) Kanter, R.M. (2005) Interview in *Leader to Leader*, Winter, p. 21.

(11) Both examples (2005) are from comments made during monitoring visits for ICN LFC™ TOT ECSA region.

(12) East, Central and Southern Africa College of Nursing (ECSACON) (2003) *Report on Evaluation of the ECSA Leadership and Management Programme*. Arusha: ECSACON and the Commonwealth Regional Health Community Secretariat, p. 47.

(13) Report (2005) after monitoring visit for ICN LFC™ TOT Singapore. Unpublished.

(14) Report (2004) after monitoring visit to Bangladesh for ICN LFC™ TOT. ICN, unpublished.

(15) The example (2005) is from consultant notes and comments from a monitoring visit for ICN LFC™ TOT.

(16) East, Central and Southern Africa College of Nursing (ECSACON) (2003) *Report on Evaluation of the ECSA Leadership and Management Programme*. Arusha: ECSACON and the Commonwealth Regional Health Community Secretariat, pp. 49–52.

(17) ICN (2002) (developed by James Buchan). *Impact and Sustainability of the Leadership For Change Project 1996–2000*. Geneva: ICN, pp. 14–33.

(18) Final Report (2001) by Regional Project Leader for the Andes region, ICN LFC™ Phase 2 Caribbean and Latin America. ICN, unpublished.

(19) Team project report (2002) ICN LFC™ TOT Bangladesh. The later Phase 2 trainer-led programs (the TOT initiative) help build up a positive image of nursing as more and more nurses use effective leadership behaviors to achieve and demonstrate positive outcomes.

(20) Reports (2003) on monitoring visits for ICN LFC™ TOT in seven countries in the Caribbean and Latin America. ICN, unpublished.

(21) Report (2005) on monitoring visit for ICN LFC™ TOT Mauritius. ICN, unpublished.

(22) Report (2005) on monitoring visits for ICN LFC™ TOT Barbados. ICN, unpublished.

(23) Based on a report on a monitoring visit (2005) for ICN LFC™ TOT Nicaragua, and evaluation data on team project outcomes submitted to ICN by Nicaragua LFC™. ICN, unpublished.

(24) ICN correspondence and documentation. Reports on monitoring visits (2003 and 2005) for ICN LFC™ TOT Venezuela 2003 and 2005.

(25) ICN documentation and experience (1996–2001) with ICN LFC™ for the Caribbean and Latin America, Phases 1 and 2.

Chapter 8
Leadership in practice: outcomes for the setting and the followers

Chapter 7 began by asking how the results of leadership and leadership development can be measured – by individual development, or by the ability to 'create more leaders', or by effectiveness of new systems and processes, or by outcomes of specific projects? The conclusion was that it was probably a mixture of all of these, and it reinforced the belief that leadership development programs are marketed by their products, the primary product being the person being developed as a leader, and the secondary products being the outcomes of that person's leadership activities. The 'primary product' outcomes were discussed in Chapter 7. Now the 'secondary product' outcomes are discussed – the setting and the followers.

Outcomes for the setting and the followers are usually less immediate than for the person. But some people expect immediate results. People ask: 'But what is the impact of the . . . program?', when it is just too soon to be able to assess impact. Indeed, outcomes and impact in the setting and followers are often more difficult to achieve, and often even more difficult to sustain. Settings such as health organizations and professional organizations must themselves take some responsibility for sustaining outcomes resulting from leadership development activities. Results that are sustainable in the medium to longer term will be discussed in the next chapter. This chapter looks more at short-term results, extending this where data are available with examples of results in the short to medium term.

Leadership outcomes in the setting (environment)

Different results at different levels over different time frames

Chapter 4 outlined some of the settings of leadership:

- *Health care organizations*: relatively unchanging; dynamic and rapidly changing; product-led (such as in industry); service-led (such as a hospital); military; government funded or revenue earning.
- *Professional associations*: nurses' associations; medical associations.
- *Social movements*: civil rights movements; the feminist movement; political movements; religious movements.
- *Projects*: a quality improvement project; planning and commissioning a new facility; a public relations campaign.
- *Work settings*: head of a hospital; senior nurse leader in Ministry of Health; leader of a clinical team; unit supervisor in a hospital.
- *Political and policy environments*: development of new policy in governments and governmental organizations and in non-governmental organizations (NGOs) including a variety of voluntary agencies.
- *Changing settings (environments)*: transforming an organization; introducing new policies and practices.

With the possible exception of 'the social movement involved' nursing leadership should produce results in all these areas, and eventually, at all levels. However, only some of the above settings, with examples, are discussed in this chapter.

In Chapter 7 it was asserted that results can often be seen more at the level of the individual, and for the local organization or professional association setting. However, as a critical mass of people with leadership skills and attitudes is built up in organizations, and as people extend their leadership activities into other leadership roles such as in professional associations and community organizations, then the greater the likelihood of impact at regional and national levels and in health policy.

Timing has a lot to do with it. People should not really expect to emerge from leadership development programs and have immediate impact in areas such as health policy. It can take time to practice newly acquired skills, and time to consolidate the attitudes and behaviors of effective leaders. And it takes time to build up networks and establish good support systems.

In addition, there is the timing of changes in the setting, such as the introduction of major changes and new policies in the health sector, or organizational development, or the setting of new strategic directions by an organization. All these create an environment of change which allows leaders to emerge, to exercise and consolidate leadership skills and to spearhead new practices and initiatives that have positive outcomes in the setting. Existing leaders in organizations may respond effectively to (and help initiate) major change. But sometimes people with different skills and experiences are needed.

Support and mentor systems are also critical for leaders if they are to sustain their motivation and energy, and be productive in their leadership activities. Some leaders report on the 'loneliness' of a leadership role. Sometimes this is because of a failure to effectively engage followers, but sometimes it is because of a lack of people to discuss dreams, goals and strategies with – people who understand all that is involved because of their own experience. Some leaders lack the 'strength' or will to call on or establish effective support systems. This can in fact be detrimental to their continued development and to potential outcomes from activities they initiate in their work settings or professional associations.

Initially, the results seen at the individual capacity-building level that then affect followers are in self-motivation and the ability to motivate others. This helps to bring about changes in the work setting over time, especially if there is an environment conducive to change, leadership and support from the top, involvement of a 'critical mass' of staff, institutional innovation and the provision of resources for change. Indeed, the two major constraining factors in work settings to gaining good results from leader initiatives are often lack of support of senior managers and the small proportion of staff involved. This highlights the inter-connectedness between the person and the setting and the importance of engaging followers, both of which are fundamental concepts in effective leadership. These points are reflected in the following example.

Results influenced by the work setting

'The training motivated individuals and contributed to their capacity. The working environment, however, in some cases hampered changes in their management practices because of resistance to change. Additionally, most improvements . . . require large-scale organizational change that cannot be made by staff working without explicit support of senior management decisions.'[1] (East, Central and Southern Africa)

Sometimes the role or the position held has the 'reach' to make a broader impact, such as leadership positions at national level, or at the head of some organizations. But people in these types of leadership position need to be credible with their followers and able to motivate followers toward shared goals.

An additional reason for some successful outcomes at national and policy-making levels may lie with the structure of the health system. For example, in some countries most nurses are employed by the Ministry of Health, while in others the health care organizations are largely separate from a national system and have their own separate governance. Yet other countries have a health system that encourages separate governance of organizations within a broad framework of national goals and monitoring systems.

Each of the above has the potential to impact on national health policy, but this potential is not always realized in bureaucratic and hierarchical systems. The following two examples illustrate what can be achieved by motivated nurse leaders at different levels.

Outcomes from nurse leaders at different levels working together

One team in the Mongolia International Council of Nurses Leadership for Change™ (ICN LFC™) program is developing human resource policies for all nurses in the country. They have started examining all nurses' roles and responsibilities, salaries, working conditions and job descriptions in their hospitals. They are working closely with the Ministry of Health (national level) on this project. They will make policy recommendations regarding reward systems that are fairer and more equitable, and consider nurse–patient ratios, not necessarily to set a standard ratio for the country but rather to determine nursing workloads more equitably in the country.[2] (Mongolia)

A team in the Vietnam ICN LFC™ aims to improve management capacity for district level chief nurses in four provinces of Vietnam. They surveyed 49 chief nurses at the district level to determine leadership and management learning needs. The priority educational need cited most frequently was content on strategic thinking and planning. The team then worked with the Ministry of Health to develop three workshops. Forty-nine chief nurses from four provincial health departments have been selected to participate in these training sessions.[3] (Vietnam)

It can take time and sustained activity for outcomes to emerge, as the following makes clear.

Outcomes can take time to become evident

'It did take time to make the organizational and national impact, but this is now happening since the people in the original LFC™ programs are now the people teaching the next generation through TOT [Training for Trainers]. It is really an awesome finding and was the vision of LFC™ when it was first initiated in 1996.'[4]

People often perceive outcomes differently, depending on their organizational perspective, or because of personal and other factors. This can occur across countries and cultures. Some caution therefore needs to be exercised when reviewing 'setting' outcomes (for example, from leadership development programs or from specific nursing projects) and to validate reported results especially where different levels of a health system are involved and when the results impact on different people. Here are some specific examples of leadership development program results for the setting and followers, at local, regional and national levels of the health system.

Results at local, regional and national levels of health care systems

Local

'In most countries some changes, often at the local level, have taken place in the domain of health policy and reform issues'[5]

Numerous new ongoing education activities for others have been implemented in different countries. Quality improvement initiatives have been implemented. Projects

(continued overleaf)

aimed at different areas of health status have seen some good outcomes and these have largely been sustained.[6]

Regional

'I was influential as regards health policies through the local nursing association, and in my related participation in various health interdisciplinary commissions.'[7] (Argentina)

'The Caribbean regional project sought, as a major sustainability and success strategy, to encourage NNAs [national nurses' associations] and Ministries of Health to integrate regional project strategies into their routine programs ... And who would have believed that in this era of declining economies, these 18 nurses could have mobilized almost $US 380,000 in cash and kind simply through understanding that they had the power to do so if they possessed the knowledge, the skills and the will.'[8] (Caribbean region)

National

'The project has been adopted by the Ministry of Health and is incorporated in its strategic corporate plan.'[9] (East, Central and Southern Africa)

'A strategic plan has been established in line with the corresponding health plan.'[10] (Samoa)

A new, national performance appraisal system was developed and implemented.[11] (Kiribati)

Effective leadership development programs will help students learn how to develop strategies to achieve and sustain results in the setting in the longer term.

Outcomes in some different types of setting

Taking account of the above observations on outcomes at different *levels* of the health care system, and according to different *time frames*, following is a brief discussion of outcomes that might be expected from leaders in some different *types* of leadership setting. The different settings were outlined at the beginning of this chapter and in Chapter 4. In this chapter, the following settings (environments) have been selected as examples of outcomes of effective leadership practice:

- Type of health care organization
- Professional associations
- Political and policy environment
- Projects

The same cautionary note applies, in that outcomes are often viewed differently by different people in different settings, and often it may be necessary to validate reported results.

Type of health care organization

In many parts of the world, many organizations and health systems have been undergoing health reform and changing from 'bureaucratic' models to more proactive, strategic and performance-based organizations. (See Chapter 1 to review this.) Leaders in these challenging change environments have many opportunities to develop and implement (with others) new initiatives that contribute to the overall aims of the changes. The following examples illustrate changes in organizational capacity influenced by nurse leaders.

Changes in organizational capacity and approach[12]

- 'A decision was taken to adopt the strategic approach . . . Many new concepts have been absorbed, partly as a consequence . . . of leaders who have learned new ways of thinking on how to handle challenges of the health reforms.'
- 'A number of organizations had enhanced their knowledge and skills in the areas of leadership, and management of organizational change . . .'

Sometimes organizational changes and outcomes come to the attention of key people who may have political, economic, personal, or other reasons to want to see change succeed. In such cases the leaders helping to influence and implement change, and the other key stakeholder(s) can become allies. In this capacity they mutually reinforce the aims of the other and mutually benefit in tangible ways. For example, outcomes achieved by one and seen as very useful to the aims of another might attract further funding. Some of this is reflected in the following example.

New skills support government health agenda

'The Minister of Health said that LFC™ had made a difference in his country because the participants had learned how to communicate so well that they helped him get the word out about the changes . . . He went on to say that initially the health reform changes had not been communicated well, but through programs like the LFC™ other nurses are helped to understand why the changes are needed.'[13] (Jamaica)

Even in countries where the health systems are still basically a centralized bureaucracy, it is possible for effective nurse leaders to influence change and achieve some good outcomes in different area of practice. The following example illustrates this.

Changes possible within a centralized bureaucracy

Significant changes took place at the local level. These were largely in the realm of quality of patient care. There were good results from specific activities in areas such as improvement in the quality of nursing care, reduction of hospital cross-infection with resultant reduction in length of hospital stay and reduction in hospital mortality for obstetric complications.[14] (Bangladesh)

So effective nurse leaders can influence change and help produce good outcomes in quite different health care settings. Although the setting can certainly influence what is able to be achieved, as has been stated earlier, there is little doubt that people with well-developed leadership skills, attitudes and behaviors, can make a difference.

Professional associations

In different countries internationally, many professional organizations run their own programs to develop people for leadership roles within their association. Some associations identify and target specific people, and sponsor and support their ongoing development. Positive outcomes from these approaches can be active involvement of good leaders in association affairs, available and well-trained people who have the skills to help influence national health policy and the retention in the organization of committed leaders able to motivate others. Effective leadership development programs should try to promote and capture an interest in and commitment to professional association affairs. Here are some examples.

Positive outcomes from leadership development for professional associations[15]

- In the United Arab Emirates and in Yemen, ICN LFC™ team projects focused on working with other stakeholders to establish a National Nurses' Association.
- Some [ICN LFC™] participants took up leadership roles in their NNA.
- Some associations were helped to develop strategic plans.

Political and policy environments

Nurse leaders internationally comment that influencing health and social policy can be extremely difficult. See Chapter 10 for more comprehensive coverage of the strategies that can be used successfully by nurses, individually and collectively, to help overcome this. Notwithstanding the difficulties, this area remains of major importance in nursing leadership practice, and leaders must develop the skills and behaviors that will help to achieve good outcomes for the broader area of health and relevant social policy, as well as for nursing. Sometimes nurse leaders in existing leadership roles must enhance and expand their skill base when the environment around them changes, as seen in the following example.

Positive outcomes in leadership practice based on new learning to meet changing needs

The chief nurse in the Ministry of Health was a participant in the ECSACON/ICN LFC™ program. She had been part of the previous more 'bureaucratic' health system, but was aware of the need to prepare herself with new knowledge and skills that were required for the large-scale public sector reforms the country was embarking on at that time. Thus she was well positioned to influence policy change. She led the team implementing new quality improvement initiatives in nursing in her country and was later invited to join expert working groups at international level. She attended the World Health Assembly of World Health Organization (WHO) in Geneva with her Minister of Health and was able to share knowledge and information with others on her return.[16] (Zimbabwe)

It is usually easier to achieve positive outcomes when the environment is conducive to change, but this is not always so. This point has been made previously. However, some recommend that settings conducive to change should be the target of leadership development programs.

Targeting environments conducive to change

'Future [LFC™ and management programs/projects] should focus their attention on organizations that are committed to change to ensure effective and efficient utilization of available resources . . .'[17] (East, Central and Southern Africa). The underlying assumption is that organization-wide decisions are required for the implementation of change, including policy changes.

Strategic alliances are another effective means of achieving desired results in policy settings. Leaders working with others in strategic alliances can focus and coordinate their strategies, skills and resources.

Projects

Team/syndicate projects as part of a leadership development program can strengthen the skill base for effective leadership practice, as well as producing good outcomes by targeting issues in the work or professional setting. Possible learning outcomes from team or syndicate project work are outlined in Box 8.1. Some of these outcomes naturally affect the team members themselves more than others in the workplace. However the following examples demonstrate beneficial outcomes for the setting as a result of effective leadership practice in teams.

Beneficial outcomes for the setting from leadership practice in projects

'Some country projects have been transferred to the Ministry (or Department) of Health. Some have been integrated into national nursing and/or health plans. There is also improved performance of those trained who are now able to discuss issues to influence the creation of enabling policies on country level nursing and health services delivery.'[18] (East, Central and Southern Africa)

'It decreased length of hospital stay, with clients receiving home care from community health nursing services.'[19] (Samoa)

If team projects/syndicate work in leadership development programs are to be beneficial and address real issues, then it is not surprising if themes emerge worldwide that reflect global issues for nursing. However, as projects also need to be manageable in their scope, major issues that are global in nature such as migration, cannot usually be addressed. Following are examples of initial outcomes from projects that reflect good leadership practice internationally. They are grouped into seven categories and cover many different countries, regions and cultures of the world. The seven categories are:

> **Box 8.1   Some learning outcomes from team project work.**
>
> - Team building
> - Awareness raising and involvement of others in the setting
> - Working with key stakeholders
> - Project planning, implementation, and evaluation skills
> - Marketing skills
> - Specific project skills such as proposal writing, grants writing, development and management of budgets
> - Presentation skills and peer review
> - Development of leadership attributes such as effective communication, negotiation, and motivation of self and others

(1)   Health and health status
(2)   Nursing and health care delivery
(3)   Nursing and health service processes and performance
(4)   Human resource development
(5)   Professional associations
(6)   The image and status of nursing
(7)   Networks, partnerships and alliances

Outcomes focused on health and health status. The wide variety of settings of nursing practice provides many opportunities for nurses to contribute to improvements in health and health status. Through their practice in these settings, nurses can impact on the health of groups and communities as well as that of individual patients. Sometimes their work is part of broader efforts focusing on achievement of specific organizational or national health goals. In the examples[20] in Box 8.2, nurse leaders initiated projects and achieved outcomes in priority areas of health status in their leadership practice settings.

Example

Dengue hemorrhagic fever (DHF) has been a cyclical problem in Myanmar. One township in Yangon was found to have the highest incidence, resulting in a high number of admissions to Yangon Children's Hospital. A project was developed involving both the hospital and the township, and focusing on strengthening preventive health education at community level. This was a multidisciplinary project involving nurses, doctors, nongovernmental organizations (NGOs), township administration, voluntary organizations and others. The outcome was a 25% reduction of DHF in the specified township through changed strategies and strengthening of the community home-based care program.[21] (Myanmar)

Outcomes focused on nursing and health care delivery. Nurse leaders can initiate improvements in nursing and health service delivery settings. They work in partnership with other health disciplines, and motivate others to want to make improvements. Sometimes they initiate training and education programs for others. They lead by example and demonstrate passion and commitment to continual

---

Box 8.2 Outcomes focused on health and health status.

- Primary prevention and effective management of eclampsia resulting in reduced morbidity and mortality in defined hospital and community settings
- Infection control programs implemented resulting in reduced hospital length of stay
- Tuberculosis defaulter rate in the community reduced, resulting in more people staying with treatment regimens
- Strengthening a community home-based program for hemorrhagic fever in a selected community administrative area reduced disease incidence
- Quality of care for asthma patients improved, reducing the hospital mortality for asthma
- Health promotion activities implemented, aimed at health improvement for specific diseases or target groups such as diabetes, human immunodeficiency virus (HIV)/acquired immune deficiency syndrome (AIDS), tuberculosis, burns patients, mothers in remote areas, adolescents, malnourished children, family planning
- Quality of life for elderly people improved through introduction of new strategies

---

improvements and innovation in nursing practice. Examples of outcomes related to nursing and health care delivery are shown in Box 8.3.

Example

A quality project in Kenya had good outcomes in the initial assessment phase, leading to concrete strategies for improvements. There had been an assertion that the standards of nursing care in one major hospital had been declining. This was associated with several factors, including internal and external variables. Some of these directly affected the performance of the nurse, and the project sought to find out those specific to middle level nurse managers and come up with solutions to address them. An assessment was done with all managers, and gaps in quality of care were identified. There was no uniformity in practice. It was agreed that the hospital needed to apply a primary nursing care focus in order for nurses to really accomplish the hospital's vision of 'being a centre of excellence in the region in patient care, research and medical education'.

First, they found that the barriers to implementing this vision in nursing were lack of resources, lack of nursing standards, shortage of staff, long working hours, lack of staff appraisal, poor working conditions, the incidence of disease, overcrowding of patients, too many non-nursing duties, bad staff attitudes, misdiagnosis of patients resulting in patients being sent to the wrong nursing units, and mismanaged referrals of patients. The results were published.[22] In their article the team said that what it needed to do about these findings is provide more training for the managers and staff. Now this hospital is a major funder of the new Phase 2 of LFC™ (TOT) in Kenya. In addition to LFC™, they are also doing workshops in attitude adjustment such as 'Journeying with the sick' and 'HIV/AIDS stigma reduction'. This project is an excellent example of how one team's vision and effective teamwork could work toward changing the culture of one of the largest referral hospitals in East, Central and Southern Africa. The project is fully supported by key hospital stakeholders. (Kenya)

Box 8.3   Outcomes focused on nursing and health care delivery.

- Quality of nursing/midwifery and patient care improved through specific initiatives
- Nurses' communication skills improved
- Application of learning to practice improved
- Community home-based care program implemented
- Pediatric service strengthened
- Customer satisfaction/patient rights initiatives implemented
- Programs and policies for safe injections implemented
- Occupational risks and accidents caused by sharp objects reduced
- Problems encountered by middle level nurse managers in ensuring quality nursing care overcome quality care improved through clinical pathways based on computer technology
- Community leaders trained and community organizations strengthened

---

Outcomes focused on nursing and health service processes and performance. Developing a performance-based organizational culture is a key component of health reform and of developing effective organizations. This is discussed in Chapter 1. Performance-based organizations usually have some system of performance measure and indicators to monitor and assess progress. Examples in hospital settings are infection rates, length of hospital stay, bed occupancy rates and customer satisfaction. Refer to Box 8.4 for examples of performance outcomes resulting from effective leadership practice.

Example

Reduced post-operative complications from 10% in June–August 2001 to 7% in July–September 2002.

Reduced hospital average length of stay from 13 days in November 2000 to 9 days in August 2002.

Reduced infection rate in operated patients from 58.33% in January 2001 to 0% by January 2002 and sustained the rate at 0% through to September 2002.

Length of hospital stay reduced from 90 days in October 2001 to 25 days in August 2002.

The main strategy was to do a careful analysis of baseline data to identify the exact reasons for long stay and to implement strategies aimed at those areas where the project team could successfully make a difference. In their report they comment: 'The project finding proved that nothing is difficult to change if any body wants to make change or make things happen.'[23]

Outcomes for human resource development. Human resource development and capacity-building is a major issue right across the world, regardless of the type of health care organization involved. Part of this is influenced by the complexity of the health care environment and by a general pressure on resources available for health care; part of this is because of rapidly changing technology; and part

---

Box 8.4   Outcomes focused on nursing and health service processes and performance.

- Length of hospital stay reduced
- Nursing care planning improved
- Waiting time in accident and emergency units in hospitals reduced
- Nursing documentation improved
- Surgical post-operative complications reduced
- Hospital infection rates reduced
- An environment created for evidence-based nursing
- Needs assessment completed on training of mental health nurses in counseling

---

of this is influenced by the worldwide migration of nurses and the need to support recruitment and retention programs as well as other changes such as the level and mix of staff. All these contribute to a continual need to provide ongoing training and development to staff at all levels and in the many different settings in which they work. Box 8.5 gives a variety of examples of leadership practice in this area involving many different countries. Often a number of quite different countries and cultures focus on the same type of project, albeit in different ways.

Box 8.5   Outcomes focused on human resource development.

- Management and leadership capacity developed for different levels
- Leadership and management capacity developed for nurses to participate in health reform and change
- Continuing education systems for nurses implemented/improved
- Country-level human resources policies and tools developed for nursing
- Roles and responsibilities of nurses assessed and job descriptions reclassified
- New performance appraisal system implemented
- Career pathway developed
- The level, content, and relevance of nursing curricula upgraded
- Potential for succession planning nurtured
- Political skills developed to influence health care policies
- Clinical nurse specialists developed
- Strategies for nursing recruitment and retention implemented
- Nursing human resource development strengthened
- Third-year nurses trained in innovative strategies for managing teenage pregnancies
- Impact on nurse retirement benefits from the national social security system strengthened
- Strategies implemented to reduce absenteeism in a psychiatric hospital
- Improved model for post-basic education implemented
- A reclassification of nurses reviewed
- Staff morale and client satisfaction in primary health care settings improved

---

Example

One team project assessed the current state of head nurses' knowledge and skills in leadership and management. From their findings, they developed standards of practice for head nurses and a training program to develop the leadership and management capacity of head nurses in 30 hospitals in the country. Another group reorganized and classified all nursing job descriptions in the country. They did an assessment with all the nurses, developed a workshop, developed the competencies needed and went back and shared with the nurses, discussed in focus groups, developed the new job descriptions and then worked on the policies and procedures manual for the nurse managers. Another group did a comprehensive situational analysis, needs assessment and policy recommendations to the Ministry of Health, including recommendations for nursing education and curricula change, nursing regulation and nursing continuing education. External funding support was received on the strength of these project outcomes, because they are designed to strengthen nursing in the country.[24] (Yemen)

In Panama, the team used the strategy of 'cascading' education and capacity-building in management and leadership, to reach as many nurses as possible in a cost effective way. Nurses who received the education became responsible for reproducing it for others. Strategic alliances were formed and a number of networks were established. In these ways a wide coverage of the country was achieved.[25] (Panama)

Outcomes for professional associations. Possible outcomes and the benefits to professional organizations from effective leadership practice were discussed above. See Box 8.6 for more examples.

Example[26]

In Jamaica, the NNA completed a strategic plan. A leadership development workshop was conducted for NNA members. A skills bank was developed and installed at the NNA secretariat. Through a strategic partnership with a private sector organization, 120 members improved their computer literacy skills to facilitate better utilization of patient information systems in hospitals and the sharing of information with colleagues. (Jamaica)

Outcomes for the image and status of nursing. In some countries, nursing enjoys high status in the community as a respected profession. In other countries, the

---

Box 8.6 Initial project outcomes for national nurses' associations.

- Awareness, interest and support developed for a newly established nursing association
- A new nurses' association developed
- NNA strengthened, e.g. membership, data base, training, strategic planning
- Communication, education programs and strategic alliances increased
- Membership increased

image and status of nursing is low. Where this is so, leadership initiatives can contribute much to enhancing the perceived value of nursing. This has many benefits, including acceptance by others of other initiatives focusing on nursing and health care improvements, staff retention, contribution to health policy and others. See Box 8.7 for examples of outcomes from leadership initiatives related to the image and status of nursing.

Example

A project focused on the image and visibility of nursing through the professional association. Despite many positive features in nursing, they saw the need to address a lack of commitment and motivation in some nurses, the public perception of nursing and the relatively low proportion of nurses in association membership. Some project activities were aimed at increasing their visibility with the general public, for example participating in a 'walk for family violence' and doing community projects aimed at asthma and breast cancer awareness. Other activities were aimed specifically at nurses, such as a public speaking workshop and producing a booklet to increase recruitment into nursing. A survey of image perception was conducted followed by a workshop for nurses on 'image building'. Networking with the media was increased.[27]

Outcomes in networks, partnerships and alliances. Elsewhere the importance and benefits of networks, partnership and alliances has been discussed. Sometimes these are for support, either for health professionals or for vulnerable client groups. Sometimes it is to achieve better results through sharing and collaboration. Both are reflected in the examples in Box 8.8.

Example[28]

A project in partnership with the military hospital focused on reducing the rate of HIV/AIDS in soldiers. A two-tier education programme was implemented, one for staff and a big campaign for the soldiers and their families. This team project was sponsored collaboratively by the Ministry of Health and the military. Another collaborative project focused on military nurses. Leadership and management seminars for all staff were implemented, and a continuing nursing education fund was developed to allow nurses to get their BSN or MS degree. As a result of the leadership development program and these two projects, the Ministry of Defence now plans to sponsor nurses for TOT each year until all are trained and to ensure that at least all managers in the military nursing core have a BSN. Both projects received media coverage. (Tanzania)

A network of students who have graduated from successive leadership development programs provides peer support; shares information regarding new government policies; shares best practices in leadership and management; provides updates on professional experiences; provides continuing education in leadership; and provides for social interaction among LFC™ graduates. (Barbados)

Box 8.7   Outcomes for the image and status of nursing.

- Professional image and visibility of nursing increased
- This was a secondary outcome of projects focusing on quality improvement and health care performance and delivery

---

Box 8.8   Outcomes in networks, partnerships, and strategic alliances.

- Country and/or regional support networks extended or developed
- Patient safety, infection control, disease prevention and safe injection in a military hospital improved through partnerships between the ministry of health and the ministry of defense
- A community network of adolescents established
- Collaboration between the NNA, general nursing council, nursing administrators and community college established to prepare current nursing practice guidelines for use at all health care institutions

---

Common themes

Some common lessons can be extrapolated from these examples of good leadership practice producing results in the setting. A few of the more important ones are:

- Secondary, or unexpected outcomes, can often result from projects. For example, project results seen as beneficial to an organization or to the health service can raise the image and status of nursing in the eyes of key stakeholders.
- Many issues are global in focus, such as the need for quality improvement in a number of countries and many aspects of human resource development and capacity-building.
- Some results are achievable in the short term, but continued effort is needed to sustain them in the longer term.
- Many projects require a multidisciplinary approach to achieve successful outcomes.
- The increasing focus on measurement of performance suggests that nurses, and nurse leaders, need to acquire skills in data analysis for performance measurement and presentation of results.

Leadership outcomes for the followers

Integrated outcomes for setting and followers

It is clear from the above examples that it is not always easy to separate 'setting' and 'followers'. This is especially true for education and capacity-building. Leaders and followers interact in particular social contexts.[29] Followers have an essential part to play in achieving the organization's outcomes, and need development to give them the confidence necessary to help achieve the outcomes and rewards for the organization. Successful projects in a work or professional setting rely on a number of people apart from the project leaders. It is their actions that help achieve program goals. Organizational change cannot be effective if the people who are affected by it are not involved. In addition, involvement in change and special projects develops attitudes, skills and knowledge in followers. This is seen in the following example.

Outcomes related to followers[30]

- Positive nurse attitudes to patients have developed
- More nurses are now keen to acquire more knowledge
- There is increased motivation of staff and greater commitment to the organization
- There is reduced uncertainty, because of demonstrated ability with external pressures and change management. (East, Central and Southern Africa)

Some followers benefit from being mentored by people engaged in leadership development programs. Others are stimulated to want to continue further with their education. Motivation can increase in followers through interaction with their leaders and exposure to the leader's vision and goals. Collaboration and teamwork improves. A positive organizational culture can develop. Thus the followers become part of a system where they do feel their contribution makes a difference. All these outcomes are possible with effective leadership development programs based on action learning for the participants and participation by followers and others in the working environment.

Followers will be inspired to achieve good outcomes if they have strong leaders that they trust and believe in, if they feel that what they are doing makes a real contribution, and if the leaders really take an interest in them and support them.

Followers respond positively to leaders they believe in[31]

'The CNO [Chief Nursing Officer] is so political . . . she is just able to move and shake things up. All the team projects are part her national strategy . . . she is a smart woman.'

'This CNO is also a mover and a shaker in the political arena. He delegates, but comes to hear the team projects and gently re-orientates things that get a bit off line. The participants love him. The country has put in [a large amount of money] for phase 2 and TOT . . . because they see the impact for individuals and organizations. They see the changes.'

A leadership development program can contribute to positive outcomes in others by extending its 'reach' to other 'followers'.

Sharing results to stimulate follower interest

Team projects are written up and submitted to the national nursing journal for publication. Strategies and results are thus shared with others, to stimulate interest and motivation to continue to improve nursing practice.[32] (Kenya)

Followers also become motivated to continue their own education through interaction with stimulating leaders, and when they see what they can accomplish with further development. Followers are also motivated to achieve good results when their activities are focused on the vision, goals and priorities of their organization or country, because they can see where their contribution could make a difference. However, getting on board with the priorities of other key stakeholders rather than their own is not always easy, as the following example shows.

Follower response to changes in priorities

The teams in one country had set their projects' focus and begun planning. Then the appointment of a new CNO in the Ministry of Health forced them to re-look at their projects and renegotiate new ones that were more in line with the national priorities of the CNO and Ministry of Health to strengthen nursing and midwifery in the country. This was not easy. However it was successfully accomplished between them, using skills of discussion founded on well-reasoned arguments, negotiation and conflict resolution. This was helped by the individual development that had taken place in the participants over the previous year. The new projects should in the longer term lead to better outcomes and ones that are more sustainable, because they have the support of key stakeholders and are aligned with national priorities. They are also being resourced with time off and funding to support the new projects.[33]

Assessing outcomes by relevance, effectiveness and efficiency

Results of leadership development programs can usefully be reviewed under the headings of relevance, effectiveness and efficiency.

Relevance

The concept of relevance seeks answers to questions such as:

- How does the program fit into the overall socio-economic and health system context and goals of the country or countries?
- To what extent does the spirit of the program reflect the concerns of these countries?
- Does it fit with the vision of the policy makers today and in the future?
- Does it meet the needs of participants and stakeholders?

Some leadership developers whose programs are well endowed with funds, and/or whose main concern is the development of the person, might be less concerned with relevance. But this should be a key concern of all parties. Certainly funders will usually demand it. Even so, if the concept of leadership as an integration of leader, setting and followers is subscribed to, then relevance becomes a key concern.

Relevance can be expressed in a number of ways. Participants/students themselves – the person – will want it to meet their needs for current and future professional and work situations. Employers or prospective employers want to know that the 'leader' has the knowledge and skills they need. Policy-makers will seek informed participation. Professional organizations will require a certain level of leadership knowledge and demonstrated leadership behaviors that match their particular needs.

Different stakeholders can have different perceptions of what is needed, or what the priorities are. Do not assume that everyone sees things the same way. Canvassing different people who may have different perspectives is important, rather than relying on feedback from one source.

Those designing and implementing leadership development programs should monitor relevance over time and make changes as required, paying attention to the setting and the followers, and to working closely with key stakeholders to ensure the programs are relevant to their needs.

Leadership practice that produces good (including relevant) outcomes in professional and work settings and for the followers, reflects to a large extent the person who is the leader and their leadership development experience.

Effectiveness

Effectiveness is concerned with whether programs meet their goals and objectives. This is easier to assess in the short term, and over a longer period some other means of assessment will be necessary, such as a longitudinal study. Those involved in designing and implementing leadership development programs will want to also design appropriate tools for monitoring effectiveness on an ongoing basis.

Most nursing leadership development programs will want to produce nurse leaders who can achieve results in at least one of the following areas of nursing leadership practice:

- Clinical leadership
- Planning and management
- Policy
- Health system improvements
- Research and development
- Teamwork and collaboration
- Nursing education

Here are some examples of leadership practice related to the above desired outcomes from leadership development.[34]

Effectiveness as perceived by participants

'I am now involved in organizational analysis for establishing a new health services strategy.' (Mozambique)

'We have developed proposals to incorporate home-based care into nursing services delivery.' (Swaziland)

'In view of the ongoing health reforms and the belief that nursing and health related education should meet the needs and demands of the society, a great deal of contribution has been made in changing approaches to curriculum development in the country. Tanzania has reviewed advanced diplomas in nursing, public health nursing, pediatric nursing and midwifery practice.'[35] (Tanzania)

These examples are from people who have been through a leadership development program themselves. So it is worth noting that other stakeholders can agree.

Effectiveness as perceived by stakeholders[36]

'It produced the expected outcomes in relation to capacity-building, creating/developing networks and contributing to policy strategy issues. In many cases, health leaders and health officials at ministries and elsewhere reported generally that LFC™ participants had assisted in planning and implementing change . . .'

Efficiency

Efficiency relates to cost. Do the results justify the costs? Was the program implemented efficiently? Assessing efficiency involves reviewing resource materials, reports, budgets and related financial reports, other documentation; talking with students and other stakeholders; reviewing communication, meetings and support systems. It also involves reviewing issues and problems and how these were dealt with, attrition and selection processes. Multiplier effects, such as training/development of others, are important – this is the impact on the 'followers'.

Efficiency is particularly important of course when there are considerable constraints on program funding and follow-up. The following example comes from a team project in the ICN LFC™ and illustrates what can be achieved within limited resources.

Efficiency in team projects

Team projects were governed by a vision that quality care could be provided within available resources. So at the end of the main project period, we asked them what results were in fact achieved within available resources. They identified:

● Improved morale and attitude of nurses and project team members
● Positive reaction from patients and greater public awareness
● More involvement and appreciation from doctors
● Appreciation from different stakeholders (local authority, mentor)

(continued)

- Awareness of the need for better management
- Better cooperation and coordination in the health team
- Improved staff motivation and behavior
- Improved use of available manpower
- Increased confidence of project team and involved nursing staff
- Improved communication and staff relationships, and interpersonal relationships
- Maintenance of sterility, ward cleanliness
- Ensured patient care and medication, and quality care
- Health education and training

This is an impressive list of positive outcomes, especially when their initial planning called for quite high budgets.[37] (Bangladesh)

Summary of key conditions for successful outcomes

To achieve successful outcomes in leadership practice, a number of 'conditions' need to be in place. These apply to all three components of leadership – the person, the setting and the followers. Some apply to leadership development programs and others to leaders established in leadership practice in their work or professional settings. Many of these points have been referred to earlier. The most important of them are summarized below.

(1) The nature of the leadership development program undertaken is important and must be relevant to the needs of the person and their organizational or country situation. Important factors for consideration are:
- the selection process, in order to help determine if the applicant has the right attitude, motivation and commitment to want the best outcomes for self, setting and others
- program design that focuses on person, setting and followers
- experiential, or action, learning, as most likely to give successful outcomes.

(2) Support of stakeholders, including:
- involvement from the outset, and on a continuing basis, throughout a leadership development program
- support in the work or professional situation (the setting) for nursing leaders.

(3) Mentorship is very important for both the developing leader and for those leaders already well established in leadership practice. For new or student leaders, it helps to guide and assist their development and also to role model effective mentoring behavior. This helps the new leader to mentor and assist others. For established leaders, mentoring can provide challenge, support and forum for critical analysis of ideas and planned initiatives. Without this, leaders can sometimes believe too much that they are right all of the time and that their initiatives and proposals will always work. Mentoring and peer review can help turn good leadership initiatives into great ones.

(4) Networking, to share ideas and experiences, and to extend the possible impact of good leadership outcomes.

(5) Organization 'conditions' conducive to the success of leadership initiatives in the setting. For example, these can include:[38]
  - an environment conducive to change
  - top managers providing leadership that supports a change environment
  - involvement of affected staff (followers), in sufficient numbers, who are committed to the change project
  - introduction of institutional innovations as appropriate to support new initiatives
  - good management of the change process.

(6) A good focus on followers, giving to the training and development of others in the setting, and involving and motivating those who are needed to make changes work.

(7) A focus on teamwork and team building, including multidisciplinary teamwork wherever possible.

(8) Planning for follow-through and sustainability of leadership initiatives.

This last point, sustainability, is the subject of the next chapter.

Exercises and discussion questions

(1) Leader, setting and followers are integrated into a framework for leadership. Convene a group of key people from your *setting* (work or professional association) and some followers. With this group, review your leadership practice in terms of its outcomes or results. Write these down. Then discuss:
  - Factors related to person (you, the leader), setting and followers, that were important in achievement of these results.
  - Constraining factors in person, setting and followers, that may have hindered achievement of your goals.

(2) What strategies does the group recommend for further progress in achieving results?

References and notes

(1) East, Central and Southern Africa College of Nursing (ECSACON) (2003) *Report on Evaluation of the ECSA Leadership and Management Programme*. Arusha: ECSACON and the Commonwealth Regional Health Community Secretariat, pp. v–vi.

(2) Report (2005) after third workshop in the ICN LFC™ Mongolia. ICN, unpublished.

(3) Report (2005) after third workshop in the ICN LFC™ Vietnam. ICN, unpublished.

(4) Correspondence (2005) to the author from the ICN consultant monitoring most ICN LFC™ TOT initiatives in different countries, based on observation and feedback from monitoring visits.

(5) Report (2001) on *Questionnaires Analysis* done as one component of the LFC™ evaluation study 2000–2001. ICN, unpublished.

(6) ICN LFC™ documentation. ICN, unpublished.

(7) ICN (2002) (developed by James Buchan). *Impact and Sustainability of the Leadership For Change™ Project 1996–2000.* Geneva: ICN, p. 16.

(8) Final Report (2001) by Regional Project Leader for the Caribbean, ICN LFC™ Phase 2 for the Caribbean and Latin America. ICN, unpublished.

(9) East, Central and Southern Africa College of Nursing (ECSACON) (2003) *Report on Evaluation of the ECSA Leadership and Management Programme.* Arusha: ECSACON and the Commonwealth Regional Health Community Secretariat, p. 48.

(10) ICN (2002) (developed by James Buchan). *Impact and Sustainability of the Leadership For Change™ Project 1996–2000.* Geneva: ICN, p. 18.

(11) Experience (1998) with the ICN LFC™ Pacific. ICN, unpublished.

(12) East, Central and Southern Africa College of Nursing (ECSACON) (2003) *Report on Evaluation of the ECSA Leadership and Management Programme.* Arusha: ECSACON and the Commonwealth Regional Health Community Secretariat, p. 50.

(13) Report (2005) on monitoring visit for ICN LFC™ TOT Jamaica. ICN, unpublished.

(14) ICN documentation (2000–2005) for ICN LFC™ Bangladesh. ICN, unpublished.

(15) ICN LFC™ documentation. ICN, unpublished.

(16) Discussion (1998–2001) with the Chief Nurse, Zimbabwe, at different events.

(17) East, Central and Southern Africa College of Nursing (ECSACON) (2003) *Report on Evaluation of the ECSA Leadership and Management Programme.* Arusha: ECSACON and the Commonwealth Regional Health Community Secretariat, p. 64.

(18) East, Central and Southern Africa College of Nursing (ECSACON) (2003) *Report on Evaluation of the ECSA Leadership and Management Programme.* Arusha: ECSACON and the Commonwealth Regional Health Community Secretariat, p. 61.

(19) ICN (2002) (developed by James Buchan). *Impact and Sustainability of the Leadership For Change Project 1996–2000.* Geneva: ICN, p. 20.

(20) ICN LFC™ program documentation.

(21) *Ibid.*

(22) Maina, P.W., Epaalat, D., Munroe, L., Omulogoli, G., Wambua, J., Wanyonyi, J. and Karani, A. (2004). Problems encountered by middle level nurse managers in ensuring quality nursing care in Kenyatta National Hospital. *Kenya Nursing Journal,* 32 (2), 32–36.

(23) All examples here are from reports (2002) of ICN LFC™ team projects in one country.

(24) Consultant report (2005) on progress and outcomes to date with ICN LFC™, Yemen. ICN, unpublished.

(25) Report (2001) by Regional Project Leader for Central America and Dominican Republic, ICN LFC™ Phase 2 for Caribbean and Latin America. ICN, unpublished.

(26) ICN LFC™ program documents. ICN, unpublished.

(27) Final presentation (2000) of team project, ICN/SNA JV LFC™, and follow-up documentation (2006).

(28) Both examples are from ICN LFC™ documentation, 2005.

(29) Cammock, P. (2003) *The Dance of Leadership: The Call for Soul in 21st Century Leadership.* Auckland: Prentice Hall Pearson Education in New Zealand Ltd. p. 27.

(30) East, Central and Southern Africa College of Nursing (ECSACON) (2003) *Report on Evaluation of the ECSA Leadership and Management Programme.* Arusha: ECSACON and the Commonwealth Regional Health Community Secretariat, pp. 51–52.

(31) Both examples are from reports (2005) of monitoring visits for ICN LFC™ TOT, unpublished.

(32) Report (2005) of monitoring visit for ICN LFC™ TOT Kenya. ICN, unpublished.

(33) ICN LFC™ documentation.

(34) ICN (2002) (developed by James Buchan). *Impact and Sustainability of the Leadership For Change Project 1996–2000*. Geneva: ICN, p. 16 for first three examples.

(35) East, Central and Southern Africa College of Nursing (ECSACON) (2003) *Report on Evaluation of the ECSA Leadership and Management Programme*. Arusha: ECSACON and the Commonwealth Regional Health Community Secretariat, p. 31.

(36) ICN (2002) (developed by James Buchan). *Impact and Sustainability of the Leadership For Change™ Project 1996–2000*. Geneva: ICN, p. 17.

(37) Final report (2002) on first ICN LFC™ program for Bangladesh. Unpublished.

(38) East, Central and Southern Africa College of Nursing (ECSACON) (2003) *Report on Evaluation of the ECSA Leadership and Management Programme*. Arusha: ECSACON and the Commonwealth Regional Health Community Secretariat, p. 59.

Chapter 9
Sustaining leadership outcomes and getting longer-term impacts

It is a major challenge for leaders to sustain their innovation and creativity in organizations facing change in complex environments. It can be equally challenging to sustain an organizational environment that continues to be conducive to change, and to continue to motivate followers in the longer term. In the same way, getting initial results from leadership development programs is exciting and stimulating. Everyone feels that things are going well. Stakeholders are pleased. The program providers are pleased. The leaders themselves are pleased with what they have achieved.

But this is only part of the story. It is not enough to define success. What is needed is to go past the initial results and outcomes and achieve longer-term impacts for the person who is the leader, for the setting of leadership, and for the followers. To see:

- the *dynamic* in individuals and organizations sustained rather than specific unchanging results
- passion and commitment – the 'soul' of leadership – sustained in effective leaders
- new leaders developed, who also have 'soul' and do not become dull or tired from the stresses and challenges of the environment in which they work.

Effective sustainable leadership outcomes depend partly on the person who is the leader, partly on the situation or setting, and partly on the quality and maturity of the followers. All three of these must be addressed if outcomes are to be sustained and longer term impacts achieved. A failure in one area could well negate gains in either of the other two areas and ultimately weaken the potential for impact.

Factors and strategies in the longer-term sustainability of outcomes

In this section the familiar framework of leader, setting and followers is used to outline and discuss some of the contributing factors and potential strategies to help ensure longer-term sustainability of outcomes.

The person

Individual people will benefit to a greater or lesser extent from a leadership development program. This is influenced by a number of factors, positive and negative, including:

- attitude to self and their work setting
- initial motivation and commitment
- degree of flexibility and openness to change
- concern over their status
- reasons for undertaking the program, such as desire and excitement to lead changes and improvements, or an opportunity for promotion, or for long-term career plans, or because they are 'sent'
- the nature of the external environment, such as health reform, bureaucratic, autocratic or democratic management style and organizational culture.

Whatever the reasons, probably a majority of people will benefit. Sometimes this may be fairly short lived, and behaviors and skills revert back to what they were prior to the program, soon after the person returns to their work environment or setting. Misuse of power, a focus on positional power and status, and a 'bureaucratic' mind-set and environment, are strong contributors to nonsustainability of leadership development outcomes. But for many, the development gains will last longer, i.e. the individual development outcomes will be sustained in the medium or longer term. Usually the positive characteristics listed above – attitude, motivation, commitment, flexibility, desire to influence change, and a positive organizational culture – that people bring into a leadership development program, will help sustain their ongoing individual development outcomes. But for this to happen there needs to be attention to the development of the setting and the followers, as well as having a number of strategies in place to support and sustain the leaders' own individual development.

Some of the more important of these strategies are outlined in Box 9.1 and described in more detail below.

- *Review, change and renewal* are critical for the individual. When this happens regularly and continuously it increases the likelihood of sustaining results in individual development over a long period – or indeed throughout the leader's career.
- *Mentoring* is an essential strategy to support change and renewal. Mentors encourage, debate, challenge and point the leader in the direction of new ideas, trends and literature. They provide support through low periods and

---

Box 9.1   Strategies to support and sustain a leader's development.

- Review, change and renewal
- Mentoring
- Peer relationships and networks
- Local stakeholder support
- Peer review and performance-based appraisal systems
- Retreats
- Formal and continuing education
- Individual development plans and career development
- Celebration of achievements

---

help motivate and inspire the leader to even greater efforts during both highs and lows. Some kind of mentor relationship is particularly important for top leaders and executives who might otherwise be in rather lonely positions. But all really effective leaders usually have a mentor to help expose their ideas to critical review and debate. Many people believe that an organizational culture which supports change and the improvement of performance, should also support a mentoring system within that organization. Refer back to Chapter 5 to the section on 'The art of mentoring' for a more detailed discussion.

- *Peer relationships and networks* are important alternatives to conventional mentors, especially among top executives, including nurses. Both have the potential for providing support and sharing mutual concerns, plans and ideas during change, including career change. Such relationships can at times be career enhancing and are another way to help sustain a leader's development, energy and motivation.

- *Local stakeholder support* is critical for leaders at all levels. It reduces the possibility of tension and conflict, and the time and energy often associated with these. It is essential to help get new initiatives implemented especially if a high degree of change is necessary and people are likely to be affected at a personal level. It provides a positive environment for achievement and success to occur, and this in turn acts as a stimulus to leaders and helps sustain their motivation and commitment.

- *Peer review* and *performance-based performance appraisal systems* are used at all levels in an organization to encourage leaders and followers to think broadly and relate their performance to the organization's vision and goals. Unfortunately, in many countries, appraisal systems are often still based on personal traits rather than on performance. These can, however, be modified or changed, even in fairly bureaucratic organisations. It may take additional energy, motivation and perseverance on behalf of the change agent(s), and it may take time, but it is not impossible to achieve.

- *Retreats*, or a team taking time out from the work environment for a few days to reflect on progress, strategies and results, can be a review and renewal strategy that is equally beneficial to the organization and the individuals.

- *Formal and continuing education* is another essential tool for individual renewal and ongoing development. It should impact on their leadership and through this, on their organization.
- *Individual development plans and career development* remain important tools to focus self-responsibility for specific development needs. They serve as a reminder that leadership development is ongoing and does not stop when a formal program finishes.
- *Celebration of achievements* and positive feedback is another effective strategy to sustain the individual development of leaders at all levels.

Participants in leadership development programmes should be encouraged to make formal plans for their continued development, and make a commitment to strategies to help sustain their development. Here is an example of specific strategies included in 'sustainability plans for individual development' in one country.[1]

Strategies to sustain individual development

- Become involved in the development of others
- Learn more in speaking English
- Practice self-assessment
- Continue study through formal and continuing education (refresher courses, new knowledge and skills, individual study)
- Further develop computer skills
- Extend business and management skills and knowledge
- Learn more of financial management
- Mentor and develop other nurses
- Continue meeting with authorities
- Get feedback from others on performance
- Be involved in nursing networks
- Repeat 'leadership characteristic rankings' periodically
- Be involved in nursing research
- Keep up with new technology
- Have regular performance assessments
- Attend and contribute to meetings, workshops, seminars etc
- Maintain external awareness, e.g. through the media, reading, study
- Keep up with new documents
- Keep informed on government plans and new policies for health
- Talk with others
- Have contact with the community (Myanmar)

Note in the above example, the references to self-assessment and assessment of performance by others. Getting to this stage requires a certain level of confidence and self-insight.

Development of language skills is identified as an extremely important strategy in many countries. In countries where English is a second language, the desire to continue to develop English language skills is often strong. This is because these developing leaders recognize that it will broaden their networks and opportunities regionally and internationally. It will enhance their use of the internet, and generally help to reduce isolation in worldwide nursing and health care services.

Similarly, nurse leaders in some countries have had limited opportunity for developing computer skills. This is identified as another important development strategy that can influence sustainability of their initial leadership development. It makes email communication possible and the ability to quickly exchange information and documents. It gives access to the internet, and thereby opens up the world of nursing beyond their town, country or region. People can sustain their development through developing others. Involvement in leadership development programs for others is an opportunity to further develop a range of leadership skills and behaviors.

Despite strategies such as those listed above, there are times when leaders find it extremely difficult to sustain their levels of enthusiasm, energy, commitment, and motivation. They can slip back to earlier behaviors, or worse. Sometimes this is a permanent downward trend where earlier results in terms of individual leadership development are just not sustained. Communication skills decrease. Little innovation takes place. The leader isolates him or herself from the setting and the followers. Some cling to positional power and status, or they begin to emulate behaviors they previously criticized in others. The organization or social movement or professional association does not move forward. Worse, the leader does not recognize or accept that the situation may be irredeemable and it is time to step aside.

Kanter discusses this in terms of winning and losing streaks[2] and the critical factor of *confidence*. Kanter believes that confidence increases with winning streaks. Conversely, it decreases in losing streaks, with the experience of failure, setbacks and fumbles. And at a time when leaders matter most – when one is trying to reverse a decline and get off a losing streak – the confidence of the leader, and often the followers, is low because it has been eroded in the losing streak. In this situation people do not believe there is anything they can do to get out of it. They lose faith with themselves and their leaders. There might be a revolving door at the top with frequent changes of chief executive officer (CEO) and top managers. In losing streaks, people have been blocked, stifled and caught in negativity. But good leaders can unblock that by investing in people.[3]

The story of Nelson Mandela in South Africa is a remarkable illustration of how one person with confidence in himself, in a different vision for a future South Africa, and in the people of the nation – the followers – who could make this happen, sustained a 'winning streak' throughout a long period of captivity. After his release and taking up the presidency of his country, he used the strategy of the Truth and Reconciliation Commission to turn around negative and destructive dynamics, with individuals and in the setting.

The setting also makes it difficult sometimes for individuals to sustain their individual development. For example, highly bureaucratic health systems that base advancement for individuals almost entirely on length of service can create a situation where there is in fact no real leadership from the top. People may be appointed into top positions very close to their retirement. They are 'caretakers', with little desire (and sometimes little ability) to set longer-term goals and effect needed changes. Worse, others in the system who have a real desire and ability to exercise leadership are blocked by the promotion system. Over time their energy and motivation can decrease and apathy take its place.

Apart from losing streaks and the more negative attitudes and situations outlined at the beginning of this section, there are other reasons why leaders do not sustain their development. They become sick. Personal factors or responsibilities influence job performance. They make an unfortunate career choice. The sheer chaos and complexity of their work environment exhausts them. So support systems need to be in place for people in leadership roles and positions. Despite these, some people will choose to opt out from leadership. If so, they should be supported in their choice.

For leaders who do continue to focus on their own development, it is useful to review what they have done in this regard, and what they have achieved. Longitudinal studies are an excellent tool for following leaders over time, to review their achievement (or lack of), and what has supported or held back their ongoing development.

The lessons and messages from evaluation of one leadership development program, after its participants had been back in the workforce for a while, are particularly relevant to the question of sustainability.

Positive attitude, involvement and support are essential to sustainability

[Asked about sustainability] 'nearly eighty per cent of respondents identified commitment, a positive attitude, and support of the key stakeholders such as Ministries of Health, immediate supervisors, nursing leaders or others. Other important factors were continued involvement in leadership activities (such as the country project, or the NNA [national nurses' association]), training and development and keeping abreast of changes, and ensuring or being involved in the training and development of others. Respondents also identified several factors that might hinder sustainability: lack of the funding, lack of support, lack of involvement of key stakeholders, negative attitudes, low priority, and constraints of time and other commitments.'[4] (East, Central and Southern Africa)

Learning from lessons such as those described above, strategies can be put forward to enhance sustainability of leadership development and related outcomes. These can be adapted in countries with different health systems, but the essence of the message remains the same.

Strategies to enhance sustainability of leadership development program outcomes

- Mobilizing financial resources . . . so as to maintain a diversified funding base
- Developing a comprehensive strategy for involving senior managers to ensure their commitment to change
- Increasing follow-up and direct support to participants after training events
- Extending the time horizon of the projects to support organizations embarking on profound organizational change processes.[5] (East, Central and Southern Africa)

Some of these strategies apply more specifically to the setting than to the individual, but both are clearly inter-related. Strategies involving the organization more directly will be discussed in the next section.

The setting (environment)

There are two important challenges here:

- recognizing and acting on how the setting influences sustainability of results in individual leadership development
- sustaining results in the setting achieved through effective leadership initiatives.

Some suggested strategies for the first of these challenges are outlined in Box 9.2 and described in more detail below.

- *Review, renewal and change.* Situations and settings change over time. Organizations, social movements, projects and systems all need ongoing review to ensure they remain in tune with their changing environments.

Initiating organizational change

'In Uganda and Tanzania . . . MOH officials used new knowledge [from LFC™ participants] to initiate an organizational change process in 2001. This was incorporated into procedures for strategic planning, which were later used in several training institutions in the country.'[6] (Uganda and Tanzania)

Renewal and change may be required, meaning responding to new influences and pressures as they emerge. This was discussed in Chapter 3 (Review, change

> **Box 9.2 Preparing the setting for sustainability.**
> - Review, renewal and change in the setting
> - Enhancing external awareness
> - Ensuring harmony between setting and leaders
> - Dealing with the challenges of bureaucracy
> - Managing the setting

and renewal of self and others). Chapter 3 also discussed the need for the leader to have external awareness, or the ability to look at how other factors in the environment (or setting) might influence the vision, and the journey toward this vision. Such factors include political and economic factors, demographic changes, new policies or new laws, health trends and issues, and changes in educational levels. Tools and strategies for developing both awareness and information about the external environment were identified and discussed, such as 'futures think tanks'; environmental scanning; environmental assessment; SWOT analysis; assessment of helps and hindrances; and stakeholder analysis.

- *Enhancing external awareness.* This helps the leader develop their own vision by highlighting opportunities and helping to identify factors that might help or hinder progress on the way to achieving it. It provides the context for strategic thinking. It is the key to the 'setting' component of transformational leadership. A broad awareness is highlighted by Ahn *et al.* in the context of organizational leadership, saying 'there is a need to maintain a broad organizational awareness while still maintaining a functional focus, as being too internally focused can limit innovation'.[7]
- *Ensuring harmony between setting and leaders.* Settings are not always in tune with their leaders. Sometimes the leadership is at fault: they try to go too fast; they ignore some of the trends and pressures facing the organization (or other type of setting); they focus more on pushing their agenda without ensuring the setting is ready to deal with it, for example in training, education, resources, or in the level of stability or change that might be required. Maybe the organizational culture needs changing before other goals can be pursued.
- *Dealing with the challenges of bureaucracy.* Leaders at different levels in highly bureaucratic systems face particular challenges as these settings are centralized, directive, risk averse, and by definition protective of the status quo rather than open to agendas of change. In addition, they usually have promotion systems based on seniority and length of service rather than on performance and the concept of appointing the best person to key jobs. They are often open to political pressures and influences. Despite this, effective leaders can influence people and help bring about positive changes and improvements in the setting. They become skilled at managing constraints. They are effective communicators and able to establish excellent interpersonal relationships. They usually have a strong sense of vision and high motivation to work toward this. They often demonstrate 'soul' in what might be considered by some to be a soulless setting.
- *Managing the setting.* Leaders who manage their settings effectively, and thus create a positive environment that also helps sustain their own individual development, are:
  - externally aware
  - responsive to environmental influences and changes
  - proactive, initiating changes and new strategies as needed
  - always looking for ways to improve their strategies and systems

- creative and innovative, not afraid to try new ideas
- not afraid to take risks
- alert to appropriate timing for changes
- able to create an appropriate organizational culture
- mindful of the need for ongoing training and education
- good planners
- aware of the pressure that rapid or major change brings to individuals in the setting.

These attributes will help bring the setting and the leaders together and thus help to sustain outcomes and increase the likelihood of longer-term impacts from these.

The second challenge, after preparing the setting for sustainability, is implementing strategies that will help sustain results in the setting, or environment of leadership activities. Effective leaders have a vision and plan for what they want to achieve. They regularly scan the environment for trends and development that might affect their setting. They initiate new policies, plans, activities and projects in response to changing needs. Some of these may be short term, but some will need to be sustained over a much longer period. Some of the strategies more commonly used to help ensure longer-term sustainability and impacts in the leadership setting are outlined in Box 9.3 and discussed in more detail below.

- *Relationships, networks and stakeholder support* were identified as important in sustainability of outcomes for individual leadership development. They are equally important in sustaining outcomes from leader-initiated activities and projects. Leaders at all levels need to involve key people at the beginning of their plans and projects, to get their input, commitment and support. Regular feedback is very important. Progress on special projects, such as quality improvement, or human resource development, or a public relations campaign, or the achievement of specific goals and targets, needs to be marketed to both internal and external stakeholders.
- *Influence* may need to be exerted where appropriate, to assist funding, implementation and sustainability of results for specific projects. Sometimes influence

---

Box 9.3 Strategies focused on the setting, to help sustainability and impact of outcomes.

- Relationships, networks and stakeholder support
- Influencing others
- Effective communication
- The concept of 'ownership'
- Transfer of ownership
- Marketing benefits and results
- Partnerships and alliances

can come from the leadership of one organization exerting political pressure to support the goals of another organization. For example, a high profile, proactive NNA can lobby government and implement other strategies and activities aimed at influencing government policy and decisions.

- *Effective communication* is central to success of projects and special initiatives. It should be regular, open, directed at and received from *all* key stakeholders, right from the planning stage of organizational activities and projects. Without this, the impact and sustainability of outcomes is severely weakened. Discussions, focus groups, regular feedback, progress reports, newsletters and e-mails, are all tools that facilitate effective communication.

- *The concept of 'ownership'* is also critical if real, longer-term impact is to be achieved and sustained. Ownership means believing in and fully supporting plans and initiatives, and working toward achieving them as if they were their own. A new project, for example, may be initiated by a team leader, but may need the full support, emotional involvement and active participation of a broad team of people. This is easier to obtain if they have a sense of ownership – of feeling that the project belongs to them as much as to the team leader, and that they can claim an equal share of successful achievements. In fact, project failure often comes from alienation between the leader and the people who are needed to make the project work. They feel no commitment or sense of ownership, and consequently their input may be halfhearted at best, or reflecting apathy and resistance at worst.

- *Transfer of ownership.* Sometimes a leader (at any level) needs to transfer the ownership of a special initiative to another person, team, group or organization, to help ensure its longer-term sustainability. Projects and initiatives should not fade away when the leader switches their time to something else, or takes on another job, or leaves the organization altogether. Part of effective leadership is developing more leaders, emphasizing such attributes as self-direction, initiative and accountability and an organizational culture that makes good things happen and sustains these positive results.

- *Marketing benefits and results* of plans, activities and projects in such a way that people understand and believe in them. The message may need to be addressed differently to different groups, i.e. personalized in such a way that different groups or key individuals readily see the benefits to be derived for them.

- *Partnerships and alliances* that support the initiatives of an organization, association, social movement, policy initiative, and similar, can be another effective way to help ensure longer-term sustainability of outcomes. Sometimes when there are downturns or priority shifts (for example) in one organization, the ongoing efforts from a partner can help keep mutual interests and activities alive.

The following example shows how sustainability of leadership development can be promoted through projects that are initiatives of one partner and funded by them, but implemented through another partner:[8]

Sustaining leadership development through involvement in partnerships

In Uganda there is a Water Project, funded directly to International Council of Nurses (ICN) by Proctor & Gamble. The project leaders are two graduates from the ECSACON/ICN Leadership for Change™ (LFC™) program 1998–2001. The Water Project teaches orphans how to make safe water and take their medications, since most of the little orphans are infected with the human immunodeficiency virus (HIV). The ICN consultant reports: 'I had the opportunity to visit one of the sites. The one I visited was excellent. The kids showed me how they get the water, and use PUR to purify the water. Since PUR there has been no diarrhoea in 7 months. They used to have 4 kids getting diarrhoea per week . . . The kids . . . just wanted to hug you and touch you.'[9]

In addition to the Water Project . . . Uganda also has money funded for an HIV/AIDS project from USAID and the Global Fund. When they start their second phase (trainer-led ICN LFC™ Training of Trainers [TOT]) they will get some of the new participants to work on this HIV and AIDS project as a team project. Basically the project teaches nurses to go and teach the community about HIV and AIDS and how to protect oneself. (Uganda)

Following are some examples of strategies to help sustain the outcomes of project work. The important factors are:

- extending the project to other areas, thus increasing motivation and commitment
- transferring ownership
- keeping people involved in some way so as to sustain their individual development
- involving key stakeholders
- ongoing monitoring
- ensuring sufficient resources.

The two examples[10] below give strategies identified in sustainability plans for team project outcomes after a leadership development program finishes.

1. Sustainability plan for 'Reduction of hospital-acquired infection in surgical ward'

Strategies

- Assign responsibility to in-service education team and existing leadership management team
- Transfer ownership to in-service education unit for continuity of program which gives good outputs
- Involve other departments: maternity ward, out-patients department, for next step of our leadership-management training
- Form a new Advisory Committee of ex-director, matron, supervisor, in-charge of housekeeping, administrator, environmental officer, in-charge security guard, in-service team with collaboration of hospital acquired infection committee

(continued overleaf)

- Get support from, e.g. hospital resources, Save The Children, World Health Organization (WHO)
- Call frequent meetings with team members new Advisory Committee
- Prioritize the problems
- Monitor and supervise the new project by the existing project team. (Nepal)

2. Sustainability plan for 'Establishment of safe delivery through promotion of nursing activities during childbirth in the labor room'

'It is not easy to achieve desired result. Project will extend to a great length of time with financial and administrative support. So our team is determined to run the following future plans:

- We are willing to increase immediate knowledge to the community people . . . through in-service training as required
- We will arrange discussion according to our routine with Advisory Committee about lacking factors, and extending the project
- We will attempt to obtain national attention to project activities and productivities for bench marking
- We will hold on [continue] our project activities through regular monitoring
- We will have a follow-up system by the expert nurses through home visit, corresponding letter and arrange clinic in particular date for lactating mothers and neonates
- Post-natal ward will be involved in project activities
- We will provide regular practice on spoken English and computer knowledge for coming nurse leaders; we will review and change our plan and policy in the future according to the areas of failure.' (Bangladesh)

Note words like 'determined' and 'willing'. These point toward commitment. And leaders generally recognize that if they are to sustain outcomes in the work setting, an emphasis on strategies aimed at both setting and followers is essential. Take the following examples.

Leaders recognize need for support in the setting

'Without understanding, vision, effective communication and collaboration from senior personnel, it is almost impossible to achieve change in our setting.'[11] (Caribbean country).

'From the project findings and our practical experience we have realized that without improvement of the whole management system of the hospital the quality services will not be ensured to the patients. So we would propose that the policy makers and the executives of the concerned institutions should improve management systems in the hospital . . . and before implementing the management systems they must orientate all the concerned persons who will provide direct and indirect care to the patient.'[12] (Bangladesh)

So benefits can be enhanced on a sustainable basis by focusing the organization in the following ways.

Focusing the organization on changes that help sustain outcomes

- Ensuring greater political support and top management commitment for organizational change
- Taking concrete actions to implement management changes, expand training and provide more adequate resources
- Improving communication with internal and external stakeholders
- Broadening participation in the organization change processes
- Setting up a system of cost sharing for the [LFC™] program
- Developing technical competency among staff by conducting more Training of Trainers' programs
- Gaining community support for development program/projects
- Networking and collaborating with other organizations.[13] (East, Central and Southern Africa)

These types of strategy can also be used more broadly to help create what is often called a 'sustainable organization', or one that has the capacity to identify and respond appropriately to threats and opportunities in an increasingly turbulent environment. In a sustainable organization, there is usually institutional commitment to improving organizational effectiveness, and a strong top-level commitment to change.[14]

Constraints to sustaining outcomes in the setting

These have already been identified. To summarize, those that relate to the setting include:

- the varying extent to which change and reform initiatives might have created an environment more sensitized to quality care and the need for effective leadership and management
- varying capacity, power and resources of different professional associations
- variations in the structure of national and regional nursing administration
- lack of political will
- lack of sufficient involvement of key stakeholders
- lack of continuing training for a core group of motivated nurses contributing to de-skilling or erosion of newly developed capacity in leadership and management
- lack of domestic resources
- natural resistance to change, often coupled with risk aversion.[15]

It is clear that sustainable institution-building – or change in the setting – requires time, a focused approach, and the ability to implement strategies to overcome constraints before they become major issues. Leaders, and those engaged in delivering planning and implementing leadership development programs, should review the various lessons and strategies outlined in this chapter, and further develop those strategies that will help sustain good outcomes for all.

The followers

In Chapter 4, leadership was discussed as involving both leaders and followers interacting in particular social contexts or settings. This is reflected in the following example.

Interaction between leaders and followers

'The team found that bringing of change requires applying some sort of leadership qualities that every single nurse needs to have, which are:

- Loving profession
- Having a clear vision about nursing
- Loving to work with others
- Listening to others
- Communicating things with concerned people in an effective way
- Respecting others views and opinions
- Building confidence and trust in others.'[16] (Bangladesh)

Note the emphasis on the 'others', not just the 'I'. Followers are essential to achieving and sustaining the organization's outcomes. Therefore effective leaders give considerable weight to:

- *Developing staff*, to give them the confidence necessary to help achieve the outcomes and rewards for the organization.
- *Motivating, supporting and inspiring the followers* so they share the vision and develop the capacity to help transform purpose into action.
- *Establishing an environment, or organizational culture*, where the followers can take even small steps and believe that their small steps make a difference. This way they build their confidence in the system, in their colleagues and in their leaders.
- *Handing the leadership role to followers* at appropriate times. This could be to assist their development, or during periods of the leader's absence from the organization, or for team-building purposes.
- *Encouraging new ideas and suggestions for improvements.* This means followers must have the freedom, and indeed feel free, to offer constructive criticism, to challenge decisions, and to test out new ideas for different ways of doing things. This will help develop confidence in themselves, and confidence and loyalty in the leader.
- *Being loyal to followers.* Leaders do not blame the followers for mistakes or when something goes wrong. They help to create a learning environment

that encourages followers to develop their skills. They coach and advise followers. They believe in them. And where followers are not able to benefit from these strategies, the leader is not afraid to discuss and follow through on the options available.

- *Teamwork.* Working with others to achieve common goals is critical in leadership. A sense of shared destiny helps make a team strong, and therefore can help sustain outcomes in the longer term.
- *Succession planning.* This involves identifying potential leaders and getting them into a development program. Sometimes these are conducted by the organization, and may consist of selected learning opportunities or additional responsibilities, rotating through different job areas, mentoring, and supporting them through an identified development program, such as in leadership, business studies, social policy, or other. Succession planning helps ensure there is a pool of people who can move into leadership positions when they arise, and contribute in other leadership roles on an ongoing basis. This adds strength to an organization (or project, or association, or social movement) and is an important strategy for leadership sustainability.

Examples for all these areas have been provided at different points in this text.

Dispersed leadership – a key to sustainability

In Chapter 2 it was noted that 'dispersed leadership' has been described as the leadership of the future.[17] This holds that there is not *a* leader, not *the* leader, but that there are *many* leaders dispersing the responsibilities of leadership across the organization. Therefore it is necessary to develop leaders at every level. It is not enough to develop a few people for key leadership positions. If organizational goals are to be achieved and sustained, there needs to be a core group of enough leaders at every level to make it happen.

Some leadership development programs focus more on the 'top' leaders or potential leaders. Some take in candidates from a variety of organizations and levels. Other are organization specific. Each has its advantages and disadvantages. Most approaches have strong potential to deliver good outcomes at an individual level. But if longer term outcomes at an organizational level are required, there are clear benefits to programs specific to organizations, or that have teams from different organizations. When these teams are multidisciplinary there is obvious potential for additional benefits.

A basic part of effective dispersed leadership is having a 'critical mass' of leaders throughout an organization, and at different levels, to be able to help follow the vision, meet goals and targets, develop an effective organizational culture, coordinate effective teams, and motivate and support the 'followers'. All of these help sustainability of individual development – for self and for others – and also sustainability of outcomes from leadership initiatives such as big or small changes in health care delivery.

Getting more impact through enlarging the 'critical mass' of leaders

To illustrate and reinforce the key messages about sustainability outlined in this chapter, and to describe how further impact can be achieved by increasing the 'critical mass' of leaders, the ICN LFC™ Training of Trainers (TOT) initiative is used as a short case study.

Case study: ICN LFC™ Training of Trainers

The early planning for the ICN LFC™ Training of Trainers incorporated lessons learned about sustainability of outcomes from the earlier programs:

- Getting a critical mass developed in each organization
- Having support from the top
- Close involvement and 'buy in' of key stakeholders
- Good communication and feedback between all parties
- Involvement of phase 1 in phase 2 to continue and help sustain individual development
- Project expansion and extension after formal program finishes
- Having projects incorporated into policy (where relevant).

To maintain standards, give credibility to the programme, and to help ensure the 'buy-in' and support of key stakeholders, a credentialing process is used. The provider organization, the program and the trainers are all credentialed and monitored through regular visits from ICN. The monitoring visits also provide an opportunity for interaction with and between key stakeholders including participants and trainers. Technical support is provided as required.

A review of ICN monitoring visit reports showed the following 'helps and hindrances' to planning and implementation. The hindrances need to be overcome, or strategies developed to work within them, for sustainability to be enhanced.

Helps:

- Motivation and commitment on the part of trainers
- Training new trainers on an ongoing basis as needed, to keep up a motivated and energized trainer team in each country
- Enthusiasm and desire to be participants in the program
- Commitment, support and hard work by nursing leaders
- Support of other key stakeholders including governments and ministries of health
- Demonstrated successes that convince stakeholders of the benefits
- Regular monitoring visits by ICN to monitor compliance with the TOT standards and the requirements of the licensing agreement; support initiatives; provide technical assistance; facilitate problem resolution; and interact with stakeholders on broad matters of program implementation, management, planning and funding

(continued)

- Licensing agreements are important to establish the contract and prevent changes based on personal factors with changes of leadership; the licensing agreement also makes the standards and obligations of both parties clear.

Hindrances:

- Unstable political situation in some countries, with frequent changes of key stakeholders requiring considerable effort in briefing and re-briefing and in negotiating support
- Difficulties in securing sufficient resources, mainly financial
- Changes in the stakeholder leadership.

The following trends should be noted:

- An increasing impact demonstrated at regional, national and policy levels, since the earlier evaluations of LFC™
- Significant local funding committed to implementing further programs
- Good success by many participant teams to get funding for their team projects
- Benefits demonstrated to key stakeholders through individual and team project outcomes; this helps secure funding
- Promotions of LFC™ participants to leadership positions such as Chief Nurse (or Deputy) in ministries of health, heads of schools of nursing; managers of health services
- Taking up leadership roles in NNAs, communities and the political arena
- Long-range plans in place in many countries to continue LFC™ through to 2009 or beyond
- Proposals to implement LFC™ in specific hospital and community settings, to develop leadership and management skills for a significant proportion of the nursing workforce
- Ministries of health and NNAs are the major provider organizations for TOT
- LFC™ is incorporated into national strategic plans in some countries
- More middle and senior level nurse managers are undertaking programs
- ICNECs from LFC™ being used by a number of universities to give credits for prior learning, and by some nursing councils for re-licensure.

These are all encouraging outcomes, with the potential to sustain and expand them through next-generation programs. In the next chapter a closer look is taken at indicators of success in leadership and leadership development, and how to determine if the money put into leadership development programs gives a good return on investment.

Exercises and discussion questions

(1) Review your own leadership activities over the past three years:
   - What outcomes or results do you identify?

– Has the *dynamic* in individuals and the organization that contributed to these outcomes been sustained over time?

– Have you yourself sustained your passion and commitment – the 'soul' of leadership?

– Have you helped to develop new leaders, who also had 'soul' and have been able to sustain this?

(2) Next, meet with a group of leaders and followers from your organization. As a group, review and discuss your findings from your assessment in Q1 above, and get agreement on the key points. Then identify the factors in person (you, the leader), setting and followers that may have helped or hindered sustainability of outcomes.

(3) Still as a group, identify strategies you could put in place to help sustain outcomes and ensure longer-term impacts.

Note: It is important that the group activities are in fact completed as a group, not just by you. This reinforces the underlying assumption of this book, that leadership is a dynamic involving person, setting and followers. Each person has their part to play.

References and notes

(1) Records (2003) on sustainability plans for individual development in ICN LFC™ Myanmar. ICN, unpublished.

(2) Kanter, R.M. (2005) Interview in *Leader to Leader*, Winter, pp. 25–26.

(3) *Ibid.*

(4) East, Central and Southern Africa College of Nursing (ECSACON) (2003) Report on Evaluation of the ECSA Leadership and Management Programme. Arusha: ECSACON and the Commonwealth Regional Health Community Secretariat, p. 55.

(5) *Ibid.*

(6) *Ibid.*, p. 60.

(7) Ahn, M.J., Adamson, J.S. and Dornbusch, D. (2004) From leaders to leadership: managing change. *Journal of Leadership and Organizational Studies*, 10(4), 116.

(8) ICN documentation on two projects in Uganda.

(9) Report (2005) on monitoring visit for ICN LFC™ TOT Uganda. ICN, unpublished.

(10) Program documents (2002 and 2005) for ICN LFC™. ICN, unpublished. The writing in both examples is taken exactly from participant records.

(11) ICN (2002) (developed by James Buchan). *Impact and Sustainability of the Leadership For Change™ Project 1996–2000*. Geneva: ICN, p. 21.

(12) Report (2004) on team project in ICN LFC™ TOT Bangladesh. ICN, unpublished.

(13) East, Central and Southern Africa College of Nursing (ECSACON) (2003) *Report on Evaluation of the ECSA Leadership and Management Programme*. Arusha: ECSACON and the Commonwealth Regional Health Community Secretariat, pp. 55–56.

(14) *Ibid.*

(15) ICN (2002) (developed by James Buchan). *Impact and Sustainability of the Leadership For Change™ Project 1996–2000*. Geneva: ICN, p. 29.

(16) Team project report (2002) from ICN LFC™ Bangladesh. ICN, unpublished.

(17) Hesselbein, F. (2004) Leadership imperatives in an age of change and discontinuity, Paper presented at the New Zealand Institute of Management Conference, October.

Chapter 10
Defining success and getting a good return on investment

This chapter brings together many of the threads that run through this book, and explores further the concept of success. Outcomes, impact and sustaining outcomes in the longer term have been discussed. In Chapter 5 it was suggested that successful leadership development programs should result in at least the following:

- The development of individual leadership characteristics and attributes that help develop effective leaders in the broad sense of leadership as we discussed it in Chapters 3 and 4, taking account of the person who is the leader, the setting of leadership and the followers.
- These leaders will have a positive long-term impact in their professional and work environments.
- The changes they initiate are able to be sustained in the longer term, or modified in a positive way in response to changes in the external environment.
- They will continue to focus on their own continuing development throughout their professional lives.
- They will actively encourage the development of others and emerging leaders.

There are many different ways to categorize indicators of success for leaders. For the purposes in this book, it is suggested that 'success' of nurse leaders (and, by definition, success of leadership development programs they may have undertaken), can be defined in ten broad categories. These are outlined in Box 10.1.

Box 10.1   Defining 'success' in development of nurse leaders.

- Contribution to health policy
- Focus on quality
- Impact on organizations
- Networks, partnerships and strategic alliances
- Community development
- Ongoing education of self and others
- Curriculum change
- Strengthening national nurses' associations
- Leadership behavior and 'soul'
- Return on investment

These categories are outlined in more detail below, using criteria in a 'check list' format that should be easier for monitoring and review. In essence, it summarizes key features of effective leadership discussed in this book. For the tenth category, return on investment, a broad framework is offered, suggesting that one way of looking at leadership development in terms of a return on investment is by using specified criteria to assess a high, medium or low return. These categories (high, medium and low) are illustrated by sharing some of the achievements of nurses across the world from different country and cultural contexts who have been a part of a leadership development program.

Finally, by referring back to the discussion at the beginning of this book on understanding leadership, the question is asked 'Is success dependent on a specific cultural context?' To answer this, any attributes, characteristics and leadership behaviors that might appear to be culturally dependent are identified, and those that might indeed be considered cross-cultural are considered within this context. It is hoped this will help guide nurse leaders and leadership developers in the way they view and internalize the concept of leadership, and interpret it in their leadership development programs.

Contribution to health policy[1]

Leaders are successful, and leadership development programs can claim success, when nurse leaders make an effective contribution to nursing, health and public policy. They do this by:

(1) *Visibility.* Being visible at the policy table.
(2) *Understanding key policy differences.* Identifying differences and similarities between health, social and public policy.
(3) *Using leadership skills effectively.* Using the knowledge, skill and abilities that contribute to nursing and health policy.
(4) *Understanding policy and politics.* Understanding the concepts of policy and politics and the policy development process.

(5) *Using relevant strategies.* Developing different policy strategies and approaches according to their particular socioeconomic, cultural and political contexts.

(6) *Influencing local decisions.* Targeting priority areas to influence such as the allocation of health resources and priorities for spending.

(7) *Participating in the political process.* Being involved in the political process and having the possibility to influence regulations and laws, and advocating for social and health improvements for the population.

(8) *Advising key stakeholders.* Advising others with power and influence.

(9) *Facilitating understanding of implications.* Promoting a greater understanding of the health implications of proposals under discussion.

(10) *Providing advice to government.* Ensuring an effective role for nurses in government departments and ministries of health, where there is access to government officials and to the political process.

(11) *Promoting the value of nursing in the policy process.* Articulating, and making clear to others, the value of nurses' involvement in the policy development process.

(12) *Understanding issues and barriers to nursing involvement in policy development.* For example:
   (a) the image others hold of nurses as a group
   (b) the image nurses have of ourselves
   (c) conflicts with the woman's role (e.g. working hours)
   (d) difficulties in describing the value of nursing
   (e) inadequate education and political sensitization
   (f) nursing not making itself more visible
   (g) nursing not being sufficiently strategic in policy development and political issues
   (h) not realizing nursing's political power, or choosing not to use it.

(13) *Developing strategies to deal with these issues and barriers.* These include:
   (a) an awareness and understanding of the nature of power and how to use it effectively
   (b) using informed position statements and marketing them strategically
   (c) positioning nursing to make effective contributions to policy such as by holding key positions in government and by being represented on policy committees
   (d) being proactive and not blaming others for nursing's low visibility in policy
   (e) being involved in change processes
   (f) exploring the relationship of gender to the level of nursing participation in policy
   (g) articulating and demonstrating the value of nursing to policy and decision-making
   (h) using formal and informal processes and systems
   (i) forming strategic alliances, networking and collaborating with all types of organizations and individuals at all levels

(j) education and training in specific skills, such as media skills (because mass media influences public opinion)

(k) making effective presentations, writing proposals

(l) timing interventions strategically

(m) strengthening the role of national nurses' associations (NNAs) and their position in society

(n) forming partnerships and strategic alliances

(o) participating in policy debates in both health and social policy

(p) understanding the value of both unity and diversity through teamwork, partnerships, coordination, inclusiveness and using the uniqueness of different groups to the best political advantage.

(14) *Encouraging individual nurses to take relevant action.* Individuals can, for example:

(a) keep up to date with health, social and public issues and develop informed positions

(b) participate in research and utilize research to influence health policy and communicate a position

(c) communicate the position by different means (e.g. write and publish to help influence opinion)

(d) join special interest organizations and channel opinions through them

(e) know who the key players are and influence them

(f) work with nurses in key nursing positions and networks

(g) identify and influence nurses in key positions outside nursing.

(15) *Encouraging groups of nurses to take relevant action.* Groups of nurses, such as nurse' associations, can use the strength of collective action. Examples are to:

(a) lobby government and policy-making bodies

(b) position the association as an expert resource to be consulted by others

(c) be alert to, and act on, health and public issues

(d) learn the most effective strategies to use in different policy processes

(e) form strategic alliances with other organizations with similar policy positions

(f) ensure public and written statements are clear and professionally presented

(g) develop and use unified positions with other nurses' organizations

(h) educate association members on public issues

(i) ensure that those who represent the association are articulate and well briefed

(j) prepare younger nurses for leadership roles and facilitate their participation in policy activities

(k) establish constructive relationships with influential people.

(16) *Taking action in areas related to globalization and health sector reform.* These were discussed in Chapter 2 as part of the background to and setting of nursing leadership. Examples of such actions are:

(a)   reviewing how the processes of globalization and health reform are affecting health and health status in a country

(b)   reviewing national relationships between poverty, health expectations and health status

(c)   promoting and contributing to health policy development in line with the health needs of the country, not on the expectations and health services of other (e.g. wealthier nations)

(d)   seeking ways to contribute to other relevant policy development, such as in the fields of labor, education and social policy

(e)   working to help counteract the negative affects of trans-national marketing strategies affecting health (for example tobacco and other products with known health consequences)

(f)   where appropriate, monitoring practices related to pharmaceuticals testing, marketing and sales

(g)   reviewing national and organizational proposals for health policies and restructuring related to health reform, and actively participating in and contributing to the process

(h)   participating in social policy development related to services for vulnerable groups (e.g. services for the elderly and children)

(i)   supporting action to reduce environmental degradation

(j)   taking strong positions on human rights abuses.

(17)   *Preparing and presenting strong supporting data.* Learning how to write and present effective briefing notes, position papers, issue papers and presentations:

(a)   a *position paper* is a formal written document developed to be read and used by a person or organization as a guide or advocacy tool for an organization's opinion on a particular topic. Those using it might be internal to the organization producing the position statement, or external persons or organizations requiring such a statement to help them respond appropriately to the issue.

(b)   a *policy issue paper* is a formal document that describes the topic or issue of concern, gives background information about the policy issue, examines the issue from a social, economic, ethical, legal and political perspective, discusses stakeholders and parties with specific positions related to the issue and those parties who would be potentially affected by the policy and/or special interest groups and their position on the issue, outlines policy objectives alternatives and resources required.

(c)   a *briefing note* is written for an internal person. It is similar to speaker's notes, to help someone who is speaking publicly in support of a policy objective. Often a briefing note is a position paper with additional advice to the speaker.

(18)   *Monitoring and evaluating.* Monitoring and evaluating to measure progress towards achievement of objectives, to document and deal with which activities are going well and which not so well, and to determine what impact on the policy process is being achieved through nursing involvement and contributions.

Focus on quality

Nurse leaders work in a variety of settings, at different levels and in different roles. Nurse leaders, in all situations, influence improvements in the quality of care provided to patients/clients in hospital, community and other settings, by:

(1) *Knowing the goals and values concerned.* Understanding the goals and values of the broader health system and how these might impact on the quality of care.

(2) *Understanding economic factors involved.* In particular, understanding economic factors influencing health care and developing quality, cost-effective models of care within this framework.

(3) *Using research.* Undertaking or using research and evidence to plan, implement and evaluate nursing and health care services.

(4) *Measurement performance.* Developing and using indicators/performance measures to measure performance in the delivery of care.

(5) *Using different models of health care delivery.* Demonstrating and communicating the effectiveness and impact of different models of care delivery.

(6) *Having a customer focus.* Having a clear client/customer orientation, and implementing strategies aimed at maintaining or improving customer satisfaction.

(7) *Assessing staff performance.* Using effective methods of performance assessment with 'followers'.

(8) *Self-assessment.* Using some sort of performance appraisal system and/or peer review to assess one's own performance.

(9) *Helping set priorities.* Contributing to priority setting and policy for the delivery of care.

(10) *Helping develop a quality focus in the organizational culture.* Contributing to an organizational culture that is focused on quality and performance.

(11) *Supporting quality improvement.* Promoting and participating in quality improvement programs.

(12) *Promoting equity of access.* Promoting equitable access to services.

(13) *Promoting cultural sensitivity.* Helping ensure nursing and health care service are culturally sensitive and appropriate.

(14) *Taking account of followers.* Leading and motivating 'followers' toward a quality and performance culture.

(15) *Embedding 'quality' in all thinking and behavior.* Striving to build a quality improvement focus into the thinking and behavior of all staff in the organization.

Impact on organizations

Nurse leaders should, through their leadership behavior, have an impact on their employer organizations, or in professional, voluntary, political or other type of organization they are connected with. They do this by:

(1) *Developing external awareness.* Being aware and up to date with factors in the external environment that impact on their organizations and create a need for innovation and change.

(2) *Responding effectively to environmental influences.* Responding to these environmental influences with proactive and relevant strategies and policies for change.

(3) *Being innovative and taking risks.* Being unafraid to try new ideas.

(4) *Managing change.* Being aware of the pressure that rapid or major change brings to individuals in the setting, and working with others to manage this. Managing all aspects of change, including the implementation of new policies and initiatives, effectively, in particular:
    (a) getting support from the top
    (b) ensuring that timing is right
    (c) preparing the organization
    (d) involving all affected staff and getting their support
    (e) resourcing the changes adequately
    (f) implementing strategies to overcome resistance to change.

(5) *Focusing on organizational culture.* Contributing to the development of a positive organizational culture.

(6) *Establishing good communication and relationships.* Facilitating good communication and relationships with stakeholders within the organization, and with external stakeholders and other organizations.

(7) *Promoting sustainability of special initiatives.* Absorbing special initiatives into organizational work plans and budgets wherever appropriate, to help ensure longer-term sustainability.

(8) *Establishing monitoring and review systems.* Putting monitoring and reviewing systems and processes in place, and making plans to sustain positive outcomes and changes.

(9) *Attending to personal ongoing development.* Paying attention to their own ongoing development needs.

(10) *Having a mentor.* This is important to challenge and debate ideas and strategies for organization and staff change and development.

(11) *Networking.* Establishing effective networks with other leaders in other organizations, to share ideas and information.

(12) *Facilitating ongoing education and development for others.* Initiating and maintaining ongoing development programs for others.

(13) *Building a critical mass of leaders.* Ensuring there is a 'critical mass' of others in the organization with the skills, attitudes and behaviors to be effective 'followers' and provide a pool for future leaders.

(14) *Mentoring others.* Helping to develop other leaders through mentoring, and ensuring mentoring systems are in place where appropriate.

(15) *Promoting effective teamwork.*

(16) *Motivating, supporting and inspiring the followers.* This is essential so others share the vision and develop the confidence and capacity to help the leader transform purpose into action.

(17) *Using position and 'power' wisely.* Understanding the difference, and exerting influence in the interests of the organization – both setting and followers.

(18) *Gaining community support.* This is necessary for community-based projects and initiatives, and for some other organizational development program/ projects.

(19) *Sustaining 'soul'.* 'Soul' in organizations includes passion and commitment to organizational goals, and is an essential component of organizational culture and development, and in the ongoing development of self and others.

Networks, partnerships and strategic alliances

Working strategically with others is a critical part of effective leadership. Nurse leaders do this by:

(1) *Forming alliances.* Alliances with other nursing, health or community organizations with similar interests can be an important tool in influencing political decision making.

(2) *Using networks.* Likewise, networks with nurse leaders and others help to extend knowledge, learn from others' ideas, get critical review and feedback of ideas, and keep up to date on trends and developments.

(3) *Forming formal partnerships.* Formal partnerships and joint ventures can be valuable in implementing projects and programs more effectively.

(4) *Fostering and developing special interests.*

Community development

Nurse leaders, and nursing and employee organizations, are part of their communities. Nurse leaders foster community development by:

(1) *Communicating with the community.* Sharing with the community ideas, information and developments about their organizations, and inviting their feedback and participation.

(2) *Being open and transparent.* To help establish credibility and support, communication with the community should be open and transparent.

(3) *Involving community stakeholders.* This is important in projects and programs that have the community's interests at heart, especially community health and public health programs.

(4) *Having good media relations.* Fostering good relationships with the media, and using appropriate media skills and strategies.

(5) *Helping empower communities.* Empowering communities to implement health programs such as for human immunodeficiency virus (HIV)/acquired immune deficiency syndrome (AIDS), good nutrition, and others can produce more effective outcomes.

(6) *Advocating.* Advocating for and with communities, in specific health policies and priorities.

Ongoing education of self and others

Some of the items below have also been listed under 'impact on organizations' above. Leaders have a responsibility to continue their own development, and to develop others for leadership. They do this by:

(1) *Career planning.*
(2) *Succession planning.* Helping others with potential for leadership, in career and development planning; ensuring succession plans are in place, and the strategies to develop successors are resourced and implemented.
(3) *Mentoring.* Mentoring others, and being mentored.
(4) *Assessing performance.* Using performance appraisal systems to help identify and prioritize learning needs for self and others.
(5) *Individual development planning.* Using some formal tool to make achievable plans for developing or strengthening specific skills and behaviors.
(6) *Continuing education for self.* Attending formal and continuing education programs as appropriate.
(7) *Continuing education for others.* Ensuring there are plans, programs and resources in the organization set aside for the development of others.

Curriculum change

All too often, nursing curricula at all levels are slow to change and retain their relevance. Nurse leaders have a responsibility to influence curriculum revision on an ongoing basis. They do this by:

(1) *Updating knowledge on trends and issues.* Keeping abreast, through reading, internet and continuing education, of all trends and issues impacting on the health sector, and through this on the nursing sector.
(2) *Environmental scanning.* Undertaking regular environmental scanning and needs assessments.
(3) *Involving others.* Having an advisory framework for formal education programs.
(4) *Monitoring outcomes.* Monitoring the outcomes of education programs, and where necessary implementing formal evaluations and longitudinal studies.
(5) *Good communication between education and service sectors.* Maintaining effective dialogue between education and service sectors.
(6) *Reviewing regularly.* Reviewing curricula and making appropriate changes.

Strengthening of national nurses' associations

NNAs are the professional bodies for nurses in a country. Many countries have a variety of nursing organizations. All should have the development of nurse leaders as a central interest. NNAs strengthen and are strengthened by nursing leadership, by:

(1) *Supporting development of leaders.* Fully support programs for leadership development, and are informed about progress.
(2) *Succession planning.* Planning for succession of association leadership by running their own leadership development programs or supporting specific people with potential for leadership through formal education programs.
(3) *Networking.* Networking effectively with other organizations and leaders, and keeping up to date on trends and issues.
(4) *Lobbying.* Lobbying for policy changes that would support key nurse leaders in their roles, such as nurse leaders in ministries of health.
(5) *Increasing membership.*
(6) *Providing education for the membership.* Developing the skills and knowledge of the membership though relevant programs.
(7) *Mentoring.* Participating in mentorship programs, sometimes those of education and service providers.
(8) *Working in partnerships.* For example working with other key organizations to develop a framework for planning and implementation of leadership development, or to support the professional development of nurses.

Leadership behavior and 'soul'

Knowledge *about* leadership is not enough. Nurse leaders must also *be*, and role model, the attributes and behaviors that make them effective and successful. They do this by:

(1) *Demonstrating* self-direction, passion and commitment in what they believe in – their vision.
(2) *Inspiring and motivating others* to believe in the vision, and to want to do what they can to transform it into reality.
(3) *Believing in and acting on* an integrated concept of leadership involving leader, setting and followers.
(4) *Bringing 'soul'* into the way they exercise leadership, that is emotion, identity and character.
(5) *Having confidence* in self and confidence in others, so others trust them and have confidence in them too.
(6) *Being a creative and strategic thinker.*
(7) *Mobilizing others to shared goals* – being able to set goals, develop appropriate strategies, and mobilize others into being energized in implementing them; being focused on performance.
(8) *Enabling others to act* – giving them the skills, knowledge, confidence and authority to do so.
(9) *Being an effective communicator* – communicating, listening to others; establishing good relationships.
(10) *Building teams* – developing, supporting and encouraging effective teams.
(11) *Networking* – forming networks, partnerships and strategic alliances.

(12)   *Demonstrating external awareness.*
(13)   *Being effective change agents* – being responsive to the need to change; managing change effectively; being able to develop strategies to work and achieve in uncertainty, rapid change and sometimes chaos.
(14)   *Being courageous*, and willing to take reasonable risks.
(15)   *Exerting influence* appropriately; exercising power wisely.
(16)   *Renewing* – developing and renewing both self and followers.
(17)   *Celebrating* achievements; recognizing the contributions of others.
(18)   *Listening and responding* to the aspirations and expectations of others.
(19)   *Having political skill.*
(20)   *Negotiating* – being able to negotiate.
(21)   *Decision-making* – making good and wise decisions; solving problems.
(22)   *Being focused*, and being more focused on followers and clients than on self.
(23)   *Achieving balance* between the different demands of work, professional activities, and home and family life.

Return on investment (includes case studies)

It is in everybody's interests to try to ensure the very best outcomes from a leadership development program. The participants/students invest time, and sometimes money. The organization providing the program invests staff and other resources. External funders often put in quite considerable sums of money. Employers and professional organizations want any people they sponsor or hire to make a difference. The leaders want this for themselves. Colleagues are often hopeful there *will* be a difference.

No one wants to see this investment of time, people, money, hope and expectation wasted. Most would like to see a really good return. Yet the reality is that there is usually some variation in outcomes. This can be attributed to the setting, or to the person themselves. In Chapter 8, *conditions* to help ensure successful outcomes from leadership development programs were summarized. They were:

- Good initial selection
- Effective program design
- Action learning
- Stakeholder involvement and support
- Excellent communication
- Resources
- Mentoring systems
- Networking
- Supportive structure and processes for team projects
- Training and development of others in the work setting
- Teamwork and team building
- Sustainability planning

Chapter 9 suggested *strategies* and *mechanisms* related to both person and setting that can be put in place to help ensure sustainability of outcomes and of good leadership practice. These included:

For the person:

- Review, change and renewal
- Mentoring
- Peer relationships and networks
- Local stakeholder support
- Peer review and performance based appraisal systems
- Retreats
- Formal and continuing education
- Individual development plans and career development
- Celebration of achievements

For the setting:

- Review, renewal and change in the setting
- External awareness
- Ensuring harmony between setting and leaders
- Dealing with the challenges of bureaucracy
- Managing the setting

For many reasons, enough of these to make a difference are not always in place. Sometimes there are some quite exceptional outcomes; other times there are a few who benefit very little; and there is a range of outcomes in between. A 'soft' framework (Box 10.2) is offered for looking at this range of results in relation to return on investment in more detail. In the related examples, countries or regions are not identified in order to protect their anonymity in what is essentially a ranking framework. The categories below are not rigid, and there may be a range of examples within each category according to different circumstances. For example, 'low' outcomes should not be taken to mean no outcomes, as they may in fact be quite high in one area (such at local organizational level), but much lower at regional or national level. They are broad categories, to help differentiate between different levels of outcomes and impact.

- *High return.* This is *high/high.* It is where the motivation, leadership skills and attributes and energy of the leader/s are high, and are matched by a high level of stakeholder and follower motivation and support in the setting, and

---

Box 10.2   A 'soft' framework for viewing leadership development outcomes in relation to return on investment.

- High return (high/high)
- Medium return: (i) high/low (ii) low/high
- Low return (low/low)

an appropriate organizational culture. Thus it is matching motivation and other essential qualities in the leader on the one hand, and in stakeholders, organizational culture (in the setting) and followers on the other. In this scenario we can expect good outcomes for leader, setting and followers.

- *Medium return.* Two broad options are discussed: *high/low* and *low/high.* This happens when the motivation, skills and energy of the leader/s are high, but there is low, or low to medium, motivation and support in any one, or in a combination of, stakeholders, organizational culture or followers. In other words, there are problems in the setting and possibly also with the followers. Conversely this scenario can happen when there is support and motivation (actual or potential) in the setting and the followers, but this is not matched by high motivation and energy in the leader.

  - *High/low* = high motivation, skills and energy in the leader, but low motivation and support in the setting and/or with followers. One outcome of this situation is that the leader motivation withers away, so there are no longer-term benefits. However, there is another scenario. This type of situation can be 'turned around' over time with strong and effective leadership. A number of books describe the experience with 'turned around organizations'. Many corporate leaders are brought into an organization for exactly that purpose. They are high-caliber change agents, and often leave for a new challenge when the job has been completed. The continuing challenge for the organization is not to lose the benefits gained from the 'turn around' process.

  - *Low/high* = low motivation, skills and energy in the leader, but high motivation and support in the setting and/or followers. In this situation, the stakeholders and followers can help buoy up the leader, energize them, and push for innovation and change, drawing on the knowledge of the leader and utilizing the leader's support. Some positive outcomes can emerge from this scenario. If not, then the leader(s) may have to be let go because their performance is assessed as unsatisfactory. This has happened in many countries undergoing health reforms, but is much harder to achieve in bureaucratic organizations.

- *Low return.* This is *low/low.* Here there is low motivation in person, setting and followers. Yes, it does happen that funders can sponsor people into leadership development programs in this scenario, especially in bureaucratic organizations. People are selected or sponsored for the wrong reasons. Their motivation and energy for development is low, and they develop few of the skills and attributes required in a leader. Often they are satisfied with their current performance and position (or status). They have few aspirations for themselves, for their job, or for their profession. This is matched by low motivation for change, even apathy in the setting and with followers. There is often a low level of support, because others in the setting see them as a threat – to the others or to the unchallenged nature of their day-to-day work. There is often a resistance to change in the setting, for whatever reason. The subsequent return is nearly always very low – or is a nil-return and therefore

---

Box 10.3   Case studies illustrating return on investment.

High return

- Case study 1: A small island nation with a bureaucratic but supportive health care system, open to change
- Case study 2: A large resource-poor country undergoing health reform

Medium return – 'high/low'

- Case study 3: A large resource-poor country with a traditional, highly centralized bureaucratic health care system
- Case study 4: A small country undergoing health reform

Medium return – 'low/high'

- No case study

Low return

- Case study 5: A country with a number of issues with the leaders, setting and followers

---

a waste of the initial investment. Usually few positive outcomes can be expected, but the vital question is, can this situation be turned around?

Case studies that illustrate each of these categories are set out below.[2] None are an *exact* fit but a *best* fit. These examples have been selected from many countries, partly because they are more descriptive of the criteria describing the different categories, and partly because there were good data available and recorded for each situation. Some countries are probably also in transition, in that the case study describes them as they were at a certain point in time, and they had the potential to move either up or down in the category ranking subsequent to the time of the documentation on which the case studies are based. As indicated at the beginning of this chapter, countries or regions in these examples are not identified in order to protect their anonymity in what is essentially a ranking framework. The purpose of the examples is to illustrate the 'soft' framework used here for return on investment. The case studies described below are summarized in Box 10.3.

High return – 'high/high'

Case study 1: A small island nation with a bureaucratic but supportive health care system, open to change

This case study describes a situation where the participants were highly motivated, but had to work within a bureaucratic system and win the support of all key stakeholders for their project, which was to develop and implement a new performance appraisal system for nursing. This they did by harnessing the support of followers, being strategic, persevering, involving all key people, and having a project they were

(continued overleaf)

eventually able to 'sell' as being in the best interests of all. They were determined to succeed, and they did. They demonstrated 'soul' in their enthusiasm, perseverance and emotional commitment to the desired outcome, and are now a good fit into the 'high/high' category.

Factors in the *person*:

- The program participants were motivated, committed, determined and enthusiastic
- They were ready to share issues and difficulties with colleagues outside the country, and invite suggestions and alternative strategies for consideration
- There was pride in their nation
- They were resourceful in obtaining funding
- They were externally aware, and used the media positively to keep the community informed of developments
- They recognized the need to bring senior nurses on board with developments
- They were committed to their own ongoing education
- They had the support of excellent mentoring, and used this to full advantage

Factors in the *setting*:

- There was a supportive chief nurse in the Ministry of Health (employer of all nurses) who, while not always agreeing with their proposals, was ready to be persuaded by sound argument
- The Chief Nurse gave clear support for International Council of Nurses (ICN) leadership work from the beginning
- Leadership development programs were implemented by the original participants, starting with the senior level nurses
- Key stakeholders were aware of the team projects and Leadership for Change™ (LFC™) program, and were invited to participate in training and related social events
- Resources applied for were generally made available (even if not always considered sufficient)
- There was a focus on the need to prepare nurse leaders for their own country not somewhere else; the focus was also on retaining nurses in the country
- Programs and projects were relevant for their health services
- There was good cooperation between the Ministry of Health and the NNA

Factors in the *followers*:

- There was support for the original program participants, for their project work and proposed changes
- A majority of the nurses underwent leadership development programs run on a near annual basis until the target number was reached; thus most 'followers' were in tune with the leaders, and the changes that were proposed and undertaken in the setting
- Mentors were chosen wisely, with advantage taken of a broader knowledge and experience outside nursing
- Everyone (nurses) progressed well with team projects despite the constraints of time and staff shortages; they chose projects aimed at making improvements in health services and implementing new strategies to deal with long-standing issues
- The community was involved where appropriate in team project work

(*continued*)

- Nurses took a positive approach to the new tool of individual development planning (IDP)

Not all small countries are conducive to and support change. In this country the chief nurse was receptive to new ideas. However this was not always the case at all levels of the nursing hierarchy, and it required perseverance and commitment – including a degree of emotional expenditure – to keep the original project on track and achieve success. A successful strategy was involving all senior nurses in subsequent in-country leadership development programs. The former chief nurse has now retired, and one of the original program participants has been promoted to that position, in an acting capacity at the time of writing. This should help ensure sustainability of outcomes, and continued capacity building of nursing in the country.

Case study 2: A large resource-poor country undergoing health reform

This country's health system faced huge problems, including under-resourcing in finance and in staff. The latter was made worse by outward migration of nurses and loss from HIV/AIDS. However, a positive environment for country improvements and regional development supported the growth of a core of highly motivated nurse leaders. The team work, and specifically the work of one LFC™ graduate, helped yield a high return in one area of the country. The decision to focus on one regional centre was deliberate, and enabled them to harness the involvement and ownership of a wide range of people and groups, including the community. This has laid the ground work for continued success and a high return being extended to other areas in the future.

Factors in the *person*:

- At least one participant in the original team was highly committed and became a driving force
- Participants reported changes in their own attitudes since undertaking the leadership development program, as well as increased leadership and managements skills; this helped them be strategic in planning and implementing their project
- They supported each other, and were supported by the management
- They were more assertive and better organized, and enjoyed making decisions and using their initiative
- They became more customer focused
- Some reported a greater sense of independence, autonomy and responsibility
- They worked more effectively with the media
- Nursing was viewed by others as important in the health reforms, as a result of the visibility and success of the country project
- The NNA believed that the (leadership) program was a source of power in the NNA, to influence policy at the national level
- One participant has trained as a trainer under Training of Trainers (TOT) but had not been able to mobilize resources for a further program; this could inhibit further progress

Factors in the *setting*:

- Health development in the region was based on a clear strategic plan, and nursing developed its strategic plan for the region based on this

(continued overleaf)

- Key areas for strengthening nursing/midwifery and allied health professions in the region included advocacy for policy change and development, capacity building for service delivery, collaboration with stakeholders, communication and information management, and establishing quality improvement systems
- The LFC™ program was supported regionally as part of an action plan to strengthen capacity in nursing and midwifery
- There was a regional centre for managing programs and coordinating with country governments, NNAs and nursing councils
- There was a second regional program related to nursing/midwifery, so the leadership program was not implemented in isolation
- The participant's project was aligned with the country's vision for health reform, that is to provide cost-effective quality care close to families; it focused on community development and ownership through neighborhood health committees, thus sharing health responsibilities with the community in an environment of severe under-resourcing of health personnel; it was also aligned with the capacity-building goal of the District Action Plan
- Mentoring, networking with health and community groups, and working in multi-disciplinary teams, were an integral part of the original project
- The 'reach' of the project extended into other programs and initiatives, and was accepted by others as a legitimate and important development
- There were plans to continue with leadership development of others, to help ensure an empowered, confident, committed and determined nursing workforce (a good description of 'soul' in this context)
- The NNA was involved in the project; this was increased after the need for more involvement was expressed
- The timing of the program and the country project was right, because health reforms were being implemented and this provided an enabling environment, facilitating the success with LFC™
- Stakeholders were appreciative of the changes and successes achieved through the project

Factors in the *followers*:

- The country project helped increase the management capacity of a large number of nurses
- Skills were developed in making presentations, surveys, negotiation, political skill, financial management, and team building
- They are reported as more committed and enthusiastic, and better planners of patient care
- Their enthusiasm is reported as coming from the fact that they were now better supported; it made them want to do leadership development programs themselves
- They were supportive of the leaders' project and participated fully in it
- There was increased confidence, and an improvement in morale
- Administrative staff reported major changes in nursing practice

In this example we see a setting where the timing was right and a number of factors in the setting provided fertile ground for success. And success was achieved – with the person, the setting and the followers. All parts and parties contributed to the success. Followers were developed and supported, and responded by being supportive

(*continued*)

and willing to participate fully and change their practice. The community was involved. The LFC™ country project initiative was integrated with broader planning and future developments for the country, and linked in with regional development. Managers and other stakeholders were positive, supportive and appreciative of the changes and developments achieved. It demonstrates that even in a resource poor setting, it is possible to achieve good outcomes on many fronts. Ongoing education, mentorship, other initiatives, a strong NNA and continued interaction with the community and other stakeholders including medical staff, are keys to sustainability in this country. However, the country has been unsuccessful in gaining funding for the LFC™ TOT, and unless they are able to build up a larger critical mass of people with leadership and management skills and attributes, there is the potential to slide downward into the medium return category.

Medium return – 'high/low'

Case study 3: A large resource-poor country with a traditional, highly centralized bureaucratic health care system

In this country it is remarkable what leadership development participants and others have in fact achieved in such a bureaucratic health care system. There were over 50 participants in the Phase 1 group alone, and all projects were centered on specific wards or units in the participants' work settings. Many of these have since been extended to other areas. Motivation of participants has been high, as it has in the setting and with many followers. Despite this, this country is put in the category of 'medium' return because their successes have been at organizational level, with little observable impact to date at national level or on broader health policy. They are, however, in the process of building up a bigger core group of nurses with leadership skills and behaviors through TOT. Unfortunately, the system for promotion is still based primarily on length of service, so graduates cannot always be used how and where they can best make a difference. Despite this, participating partners in the LFC™ programs make a determined effort to include 'graduates' wherever possible on national committees and in further training opportunities. Political allegiances in the country are divisive and contribute to divisiveness within nursing. Health reform is on the agenda, but slow to happen. Thus there are many challenges to be met, but we believe this country has the clear potential to move into the high return category. We hope to see this happen in the near future as developments and achievements become consolidated, and impacts are extended from local to regional and national level.

Factors in the *person*:

- Participants were motivated, enthusiastic and committed to making improvements; where motivation for some was lower at the beginning, this increased as they grew in confidence with demonstrated successes and good project outcomes
- They were proud of their country
- They accepted the reality of a resource-poor setting and showed determination to make improvements within financial constraints
- Although sometimes hampered by personal or family crisis and politically invoked strife, the project teams persevered and compensated for periods of low activity on behalf of some team members

(continued overleaf)

- Participants developed confidence and skills, and through this became empowered in a health system where nursing did not have a high image
- A number of participants undertook further education
- There was a desire to increase computer skills and be able to use email and the internet, to increase the potential for information and networking outside the country
- They became more confident in interaction with 'higher authority' in hospital settings
- They nearly all demonstrated personal growth and development of leadership attitudes, skills and behaviors
- Nearly a dozen nurses in this country-focused LFC™ program have trained as trainers under TOT

Factors in the *setting*:

- The health system was a highly centralized bureaucracy; the nursing section in the Department of Health (in the centre) controlled all nursing personnel including appointments and transfers of all senior staff
- Promotion of nurses was based mainly on length of service; this did not always ensure the 'right' person was appointed to leadership positions; however there was good opportunity for nurses to exercise leadership at a clinical level, which the LFC™ people did
- The central Division of Nursing and the country's World Health Organization (WHO) office were partners with ICN in the LFC™ program, and gave their expertise, time and support to hospital teams throughout the program and subsequently with TOT-led programs
- WHO and the Department of Health mobilized funds for ongoing TOT-led programs, thus building up a core of people in selected organizations with leadership and management skills
- There was good interdisciplinary teamwork, and excellent support from medical and managerial staff at the local organizational level
- Stakeholders in the organizations supported team project work and in many cases enabled the mobilization of additional resources
- The political environment in the country was at times de-stabilizing, with strikes, shootings, and factionalism
- There were frequent changes of leadership at the top of organizations and in the Department of Health; this contributed to slow change in the health system environment
- The NNA was small, and not well organized; there are however indications of change and a more strategic direction being established
- Relationships between key nursing organizations/leaders were not very effective

Factors in the *followers*:

- Many nurses had limited opportunities for further education and promotion
- This, together with working conditions, the image of nursing and other factors, helped create a general apathy among many nursing staff
- Where the LFC™ participants implemented team projects, this apathy often turned to enthusiasm and motivation for further education and for effecting quality improvements in care

(*continued*)

- A range of staff from different disciplines were involved in team projects (most projects were in hospital settings and related in some way to improvement in quality of care)

As stated earlier, it was remarkable what followers, leaders and other stakeholders were able to accomplish in such a difficult setting. In some ways the 'medium' return on investment for this country is unfair, because some of the outcomes have indeed been excellent. Certainly personal motivation and desire for improvements are fairly widespread. In many ways this country is in transition from 'medium' to 'high'. If current good outcomes are able to be sustained in the longer term, given the general environment and the need for further changes in it, and if nursing is able to extend its impact to regional and national levels with greater involvement in health policy directions for the country, they would indeed be able to justify a classification of high return on investment.

Case study 4: A small country undergoing health reform

This example is of a small country where the motivation of LFC™ participants was very high, and some excellent outcomes were achieved. However, the full potential to achieve a high return has not yet been realized, partly because of other personal and professional demands on participants, and partly because of issues in relationships between different people and groups.

Factors in the *person*:

- One participant had a much higher profile than the others, and was promoted and utilized in a number of different areas where her skills did contribute to good outcome; however this left her with more limited time and energy to devote to other nursing development activities
- The other participants were less visible on the national scene, for different reasons relating partly to their circumstances and partly to other factors
- All participants achieved personal growth and leadership development as a result of their involvement in LFC™
- One participant has trained as a trainer for LFC™ TOT, but the program was slow to get started

Factors in the *setting*:

- The environment was conducive to change and there was an active health reform program
- In the earlier days of the health reform program there appeared to be minimal consultation with a range of stakeholder groups; it was driven by a smaller team
- More latterly, the NNA was formally invited by government to give input into policies and decisions
- Collaboration was established with nongovernmental organizations (NGOs)
- There were numerous changes in key stakeholders in government, in the NNA, and other organizations, but the team project 'survived' these changes
- Stakeholders in the setting were motivated and supportive of the LFC™ country team project; subsequent support for the TOT initiative varied among stakeholders, and TOT was slow to get off the ground but finally made it

(continued overleaf)

- The NNA was initially very supportive, and was strengthened by some of the LFC™ activities; this support later waned as personal differences emerged
- A range of positive outcomes have been achieved, but the full potential is not yet realized

Factors in the *followers*:

- A number of nurses have benefited from an earlier leadership development program implemented by LFC™ participants as part of their country team project
- Nurses have shown support for further leadership development through TOT
- Initially nurses did not buy in to the project; the use of negotiation and political skills helped to overcome this

So in this example, the person, setting and followers were generally all conducive to a high level of outputs and achievement. Much has in fact been achieved. A more concerted team approach, perhaps more aggressive marketing, better teamwork and support of different nursing leaders, and an ongoing LFC™ TOT initiative, could help move this country into the high return category.

Medium return – 'low/high'

ICN has no case studies from the LFC™ which would adequately reflect this situation, largely because where motivation for some people may be low, especially at the beginning of a program, this is usually a reflection of low motivation and enthusiasm in the setting. This does not lead to high outputs in the LFC™ program, based as it is on action learning in the work setting.

Low return – 'low/low'

Case study 5: A country with a number of issues with the leaders, setting and followers

In this country, the LFC™ participants had reasonably high motivation, at least initially. However this was not high enough, nor were their leadership skills sufficiently strong to develop strategies that would counter the negative features in the setting and enable them to access the structures that would provide support and help promote their team project. The focus of the team project became lost as the team's energies were directed at solving issues in its implementation, So this country is classified in the low return group – indeed, one of the few in the whole ICN LFC™ experience.

Factors in the *person*:

- Motivation ebbed and flowed; in fact the participants stopped work on country activities for about six months in order to gather their forces together, as they said it was very hard to find support anywhere despite knocking on several doors and lobbying for support
- Participants found it difficult to develop a clear, integrated country project; rather they tended to work on specific activities that they tried to articulate to the 'power structures' in nursing; thus some people found it hard to understand what they

(continued)

were doing that was different from current activities; there were tensions between some nurses and groups

- There was some observable individual growth, confirmed by direct supervisors
- There was personal growth and support gained though working with their mentor
- They initiated some new developments and improvements in their immediate work environments
- Generally they could be described as low on 'soul'
- Participants did not involve themselves in training for TOT

Factors in the *setting*:

- The broader political environment in the country was unstable, with many changes of directors of health and a lack of direction regarding health sector reform; so work with previous politicians and health directors was lost when these changed
- The nurses' association was weak, with many changes in leadership and a low membership
- Some innovations (this confirmed by direct supervisors) in the their working environment were implemented by participants, but there was little or no apparent impact at country level such as with the nurses' association, the Ministry of Health and teaching institutions
- Key stakeholders reported very little information about the LFC™ or the country project, suggesting a low visibility of the participants, or lack of sufficient communication between them and key others, or lack of interest to take in information they were given and find out more
- There was no commitment from the Ministry of Health and teaching institutions to the LFC™, and the participants said they received no support
- Stakeholders acknowledged a lack of economic resources, and that those available were currently engaged elsewhere
- Improving leadership capacity in a changing environment was acknowledged by others as important; but this did not extend to clear support for these participants and their project
- There appeared to be weak nursing leadership at national level, and differences of opinion as to who should 'own' leadership development, i.e. where it should be placed
- Some key stakeholders commented that they ignored the project because they had not participated in it
- A long-standing human resource development for nursing project in the Ministry of Health, had reportedly blocked access to that structure for the LFC™ participants
- There were consistent reports of an autocratic nursing leadership in the Ministry of Health, with centralized resources and limited participation of others
- The strength and credibility of nursing in the country is low

Factors in the *followers*:

- Benefits of LFC™ were said by some to be for the participants only, with little flow-on to others
- There were some training and development activities for others, implemented by the participants
- There was generally low participation in the participant's project, and a low 'reach'

(continued overleaf)

- Nurses in the country were reported as being very divided, with lack of coordination of nursing projects generally
- Nursing interest is hard to get because of lack of time and energy, with somewhere around 90% working in two or three jobs to help improve their low income
- There are about 90 nursing assistants to every 10 nurses
- Because of the frequent changes of government, nurses were reportedly more interested in protecting their positions than in working for a common project

This is an example of nurses in a leadership development program working in a difficult country context. Apart from at a personal level, few outcomes were perceived by others from project activities in the country. It is clear that in order to have achieved more, they needed to address factors in the setting. Perhaps some of the following strategies might have helped:

- Wide marketing of their activities and project to a range of key stakeholders
- Finding a 'home' for the project, to help lend it credibility, to provide support and to provide a negotiating base for resources and acceptance by others
- Having a more clearly defined project they could describe and explain to others in relation to identifiable goals and targets
- Working with the NNA to help strengthen it and increase membership
- Communicating with all key stakeholders on an ongoing basis
- Identifying early the potential areas of support, and also the anticipated hindrances, and developing a strategic plan to harness the support and deal with the hindrances. As it was, without this strategic approach, events kept emerging over time to the extent they finally became overwhelming

Some factors were clearly outside their control, such as the unstable political environment and frequent changes of key players in the health system. This puts extra demands on nurse leaders as they need to be constantly briefing and re-briefing. It is a good example of how some situations demand that much extra skill in external awareness and environmental assessment, and in strategic thinking and planning. This can help increase the 'return on investment' in 'low/low' situations such as described here.

Is success dependent on a specific cultural context?

In other words, does culture help determine success? This question was asked at the beginning of this book. It can now be said that specific attributes, characteristics or leadership behaviors that might appear to be directly linked to the culture of the leader's country have not been identified. There are of course numerous factors from specific cultures that will influence leadership behavior, but interestingly these are often common in different cultures and are usually more related to the structure and stage of development of the society and its health system. Here are some examples of factors expressed in many different cultures and societies that could influence the development of nursing leadership:

- A low image and status of nursing
- The status of women
- A bureaucratic, highly centralized health system

- Low resources given to nursing
- Poor access to continuing education
- Unstable political environment.

So people might say, for example, 'Women are not accepted by men as leaders in our culture'. Whereas the real issue often seemed to center around confidence in self. Or they might say 'It's not in our culture to put ourselves forward, or to speak up in front of others'. Again, this often related to confidence. Growth in confidence comes up time and again as one of the most frequently occurring areas of development in the ICN leadership development programs. This is based on a wide variety of action-learning situations in the classroom and in the work environment. Positive feedback from others and the achievement of good outcomes was a significant contributor to the development of confidence. With this growth, people can see what they are capable of achieving, and 'culture' is often then seen more as an excuse, and usually discarded.

A bureaucratic health care system also contributes to behaviors of leaders that some attribute to culture. 'Bossiness' for example, and 'giving orders' or focusing on rigid rules and procedures. Such systems still exist in many different cultures, and tend by their nature to generate certain types of behaviors. These behaviors usually relate more to the type of organizational or work setting than to the culture of the country.

An unstable political environment in a number of countries often had a flow-on effect to health and nursing leadership that is sometimes said to be 'part of our culture'. Yet, the same unstable political situation appears in many different countries and cultures, and the impacts on nursing are often similar.

In Chapter 2 it was said that the ICN LFC™ experience, which crosses many different country and cultural boundaries and settings, showed some consistent results despite widely different political, economic and cultural settings. This is reiterated again now, and attributed to the 'action-learning' methodology within those settings, as well as adaptation of program content to the different environments. These allowed the development of realistic strategies for dealing with issues in both the short and the longer term. So, while the issues might be different or expressed differently, the leadership behaviors needed for dealing with them are usually the same.

There are always some examples that may appear to be obvious exceptions. Take the following.

Traditional or cultural?

'In Africa [at least in this country] it is not frequent to hear the vocabularies of justice, fidelity, honesty. Someone rich is given great importance without questioning anything . . .' (In fact, we could say that similar values exist in some segments of a number of other non-African countries.) And the following description of management style (said to be culturally related) from the same country is also familiar in traditional bureaucracies in a number of countries in other parts of the world.

(continued overleaf)

'There is no spirit of strategic programming; they are less committed to their work; there is a high willingness to be praised because of his position, not for what he does; he doesn't value the work of subordinates; the talents of subordinates are not used because [the leader] doesn't want to be overcome by his subordinate; he is highly preoccupied with his own satisfaction; he doesn't care about client satisfaction.'[3]

However, two further items on this list, which could be culturally related, were: 'It is the chief who knows everything; there is a blacklist of workers who are shown to be intelligent'. However, neither of these are common attributes of leadership as we have defined it.

This example sounds more like a traditional bureaucratic management system in a highly traditional country, still influenced by the power of the chiefs. Compare it with the experiences of other countries in the region, described in examples elsewhere in this book. (Country in Africa)

There are other cultures where family or ethnic patronage has an impact in areas such as appointments and staff/work practices. Thus these situations might dictate *who* the leader will be, but not necessarily *how* he/she will or should lead. Similarly in some societies, students listen but do not readily ask questions or spontaneously offer comments. They might say this is because of their culture, whereas often it is because of the type of education experience they have had in their schools since childhood.

For the most part, the LFC™ experience has found that learning activities developed for the program were able to be comfortably applied across all cultures and country settings. But factors external to the program content, such as how to meet and greet people, or seat them in official functions, or what to wear, or when to break for prayers, were done in accordance with cultural mores. The key learning here is that it is important to adapt leadership knowledge, attributes and behaviors to different cultural contexts, especially in the design and implementation of a leadership development program. However, it is wise to remember that a leader is a leader is a leader . . .

There are an enormous variety of leaders for as wide a variety of settings and of groups of followers. Style will be different. Some behaviors and skills will be needed more in some types of settings than in others. Followers may require different skills and attributes in their leaders according to setting, type of organization, the nature and timing of change, political and social factors in the broader environment, and a number of other factors.

What is needed, then, is for leaders and leadership developers to be knowledgeable and experienced; to be able to adapt to different settings and situations; to be flexible in their thinking and leadership behavior; and to be wary about using 'labels' – like 'culture' – to explain differences that may or may not be relevant.

Exercises and discussion questions

(1) How many of the ten categories of 'success' apply to your own leadership practice?

(2) One of the important categories of success for a nurse leader is contribution to health policy. Review your own leadership practice against each of the 18 criteria. Write down some strategies to address any areas that need strengthening.

(3) With a group of leaders in your own organization, discuss the categories for return on investment, and identify (with justification) where your organization best fits. Use this information to plan for further leadership development for identified personnel.

(4) Celebrating achievements, and recognizing the contributions of others, is one of the criteria listed under the category 'leadership behavior and soul'. Do you do enough to celebrate achievements, and recognize others, in your leadership practice? Discuss with others their ideas for doing more, and make concrete plans to put good ideas into action.

References and notes

(1) This section on policy is mainly adapted from ICN (2005) Health Policy Package. Geneva. ICN. This package (the ICN HPP) draws upon different ICN and other documents to present a teaching-learning resource that can be used by groups to help develop knowledge and skills in the policy process. It contains information, slides and group activities, and is available from ICN.

(2) All case studies are developed from ICN LFC™ data and documentation. ICN, unpublished.

(3) Participant written report (2001) in the ECSACON/ICN LFC™. ICN, unpublished.

Chapter 11
Making a difference

The development of nursing leadership is critical to the future of health services across the world. Nursing can make a difference. If enough nurses develop their leadership capacity, then nursing leadership can impact at all levels and in many different sectors of the health services. Effective nursing leadership can impact on health policy at all levels. It can help maintain high standards of care in different clinical settings. It can benefit patients and communities by contributing to wise priority setting and effective use of available resources.

At the beginning of this book, the complexity of health services in change was discussed, and the implications for nursing leadership outlined. To make a difference, the leadership behavior of individuals, and of nurses collectively, is equally important. And both aspects of leadership have the integrated components of leader, setting, and followers. This book has focused on what makes a leader, how to prepare them in leadership development programs, and how to assess their success, or effectiveness.

To look at leaders individually, it is necessary to be clear on who is being referred to by the term 'leader'. The concept of 'dispersed leadership' is used in this book as the leadership of the future.[1] This holds that there is not *a* leader, not *the* leader, but that there are *many* leaders dispersing the responsibilities of leadership across the organization. Gone are up/down, top/bottom, superior/subordinate relationships. We must be developing leaders at every level. So leaders are certainly not only those who occupy the positions at the top of an organization. Leadership is not about position or about charisma, and these do not guarantee that the person behaves as a leader. Leadership – leadership skills and behaviours – can be learned.

Many countries have been involved in nursing leadership development for a long time. Sometimes this has focused on positional leadership, and has not been generally accessible to a larger number of nurse leaders at different levels and in many different situations. However, other countries have consciously made leadership development opportunities available to larger numbers of nurses, thus helping to ensure a 'critical mass' of leaders for the complex and rapidly changing world of health care systems today. The preparation of nurse leaders often yields visible results at individual level quite quickly. Skills and attributes become apparent in people's leadership behavior, and develop more with ongoing experience. Nurse leaders can exert leadership, inspiring and motivating others toward the achievement of a vision or of specific goals held in common. This is often particularly visible in work or professional environments.

However, the impact of nursing leadership on a broader level is usually dependent on the 'critical mass' of nurses and nurse leaders working collectively toward common goals. Countries that are now aiming to prepare nurse leaders in greater numbers than previously, recognizing the importance of 'dispersed leadership', must make available a variety of opportunities for leadership development. On their leadership development journeys, countries must also stay focused on their long-term vision. Usually this is related in some way to making a difference.

Leadership development aimed at making a difference on a broad scale is a long-term strategy, and can yield results at country and policy levels slowly. But working together, nurses can make a difference. Partnerships and strategic alliances have been discussed in this book as a means for organizations with a different focus to harness their goals in common, and work together in specific circumstances for a common purpose. Collectively, more can be achieved, whether it is a leader working with followers, or the leadership of different organizations working together in formal or informal partnerships.

Leadership can be a way of thinking, a way of behaving, a way of being. Indeed, as noted earlier, Norton and Smythe have reminded us that seeking a prescriptive leadership formula is 'like trying to pick up mercury with your fingers . . . as soon as you think you've got it, you've lost it'.[2] But ideas and understanding of leadership, rather than a prescriptive formula, are there to guide and empower us. This book should help do this for you.

Exercises and discussion questions

(1) Write down how you see your leadership role. What specific leadership attributes and behaviors do you use most? What need to be developed further?
(2) List your long-term goals as a nurse leader. Break these down into specific shorter-term objectives, and develop a plan with strategies and timeline for each of the key areas you have identified.
(3) If you are serious about your career goals and do not yet have a mentor, get one!
(4) Discuss your career plans with your mentor. Make any adjustments. Then act!

References and notes

(1) Hesselbein, F. (2004) Leadership imperatives in an age of change and discontinuity. Paper presented at the New Zealand Institute of Management Conference, October, pp. 2–3.
(2) Norton, A. and Smythe, L. (2005) *Not Just Another Book About Leadership*. Pre-publication draft, pp. 9–10. Quoted with permission of the authors.

Abbreviations and glossary

Buy-in
Belief in, and commitment of specified people or groups to something

CEO
Chief Executive Officer

CNO
Chief Nursing Officer

ECSA
East, Central and Southern Africa

ECSACON
East, Central and Southern Africa College of Nursing

ECSACON/ICN LFC™
Formal joint venture between ECSACON and ICN to deliver the LFC™ program

Funders
Individuals, associations or organizations that provided funding support for LFC™ projects and programs, or part(s) thereof

ICN
International Council of Nurses

ICN LFC™ Evaluation
Evaluation of LFC™ programs 1996–2000, consisting of four components: documents analysis; questionnaires; country case studies; and longitudinal study. The first three components were undertaken between 2000 and 2001, and focused on the early programs completed between 1997 and 2000, before the Training of Trainers (TOT) commenced. This provided data for planning TOT and its resources. The longitudinal study (fourth component) is ongoing.

ICN HPP
ICN Health Policy Package, 2005

ICNECs
International Continuing Nursing Education Credits, issued by ICN

IDP
Individual development plan, a structured learning tool used in the ICN LFC™

JV
Joint venture

KRA
Key Result Area

LFC™
Leadership for Change™. An action-learning leadership development program to develop nurses as effective leaders and managers in a constantly changing health environment. Developed and copyrighted by ICN and implemented since 1996.

MA
Master of Arts

Mentee
Person being mentored by another

MOH
Ministry of Health

Monitoring visits
Visits made to countries implementing LFC™ TOT programs, to ensure they comply with standards and criteria set out in the Agreements, and to provide assistance and technical support as needed

NGO
Nongovernmental organization

NNA
National nurses' association

OECD
Organization for Economic Co-operation and Development

Ownership [of LFC™]
A group or organization that accepts responsibility for all or some aspects of LFC™ delivery

Participants
Students in the ICN LFC™ program

Provider Organization
The organization credentialed by ICN to provide the LFC™ program with certified trainers under the ICN LFC™ TOT initiative

REDSO
Regional Economic Development Services for East and Southern Africa

RPL
Recognition of prior learning

SNA/ICN LFC™
Formal JV between the Singapore Nurses Association and ICN to deliver the LFC™ program

Stakeholders [LFC™]
Those individuals or groups who influence, or are influenced by, something. For example, those who have an interest in the outcomes of a program and work with it and support it in some way

TOT
Training of Trainers

USAID
US Agency for International Development

WHO
World Health Organization

> **SEARO**
> WHO South East Asia Regional Office
>
> **AFRO**
> WHO Africa Regional Office
>
> **PAHO**
> WHO Pan American Health Organization
>
> **EMRO**
> WHO Eastern Mediterranean Regional Office
>
> **EURO**
> WHO European Regional Office
>
> **WPRO**
> WHO Western Pacific Regional Office

UAE
United Arab Emirates

UK
United Kingdom

US
United States [of America]

UNCTAD
United Nations Conference on Trade and Development

UNDP
United Nations Development Programme

References

There is a huge literature on leadership covering many different aspects and fields. A comprehensive literature review is not included in this book, and only those specific references used in the text are listed below. A large number of text references are from ICN documentation, and for the purposes of this list of references these have mainly been grouped under 'ICN: Documents for the Leadership for Change™ program, 1996–2005'. Some of these were written by participants. Others were written by mentors, national coordinators, regional project leaders and other stakeholders. And some were written by consultants contracted by ICN and by ICN staff.

American spelling has been used throughout the text, but where references use English spelling, this is retained in the footnotes and references.

Ahn, M.J., Adamson, J.S. and Dornbusch, D. (2004) From leaders to leadership: managing change. *Journal of Leadership and Organizational Studies*, 10 (4), 114.

Anderson, R.A., Issel, L.M. and McDaniel, R.R. (2003). Nursing homes as complex adaptive systems: relationship between management practice and resident outcomes. *Nursing Research*, 52 (1), 12–21.

Appleby, D. (1999) Choosing a Mentor. Available at: http://www.psichi.org/pubs/articles/article_107.asp (August 21).

Bennis. W. and Nanus, B. (1985) *Leaders: The Strategies for Taking Charge*. New York: Harper and Row.

Bethel, S.M. (1990) *Making a Difference: 12 Qualities That Make You a Leader*. New York: Berkley Books.

Bethel, S.M. (1993) *Beyond Management to Leadership: Designing the 21st Century Association*. Foundation of the American Society of Association Executives.

Burns, J.P. (2001), Complexity science and leadership in health care. *Journal of Nursing Administration*, 31 (10), 474–482.

Cammock, P. (2003) *The Dance of Leadership: The Call for Soul in 21st Century Leadership*. Auckland: Prentice Hall Pearson Education in New Zealand Ltd.

Champy, J. (1995) *Re-engineering Management: the Mandate for New Leadership*. UK: Harper Collins.

Drucker, P. (1992) *Managing for the Future: The 1990s and Beyond*. New York: Truman Talley Books.

Duck, J.D. (1993) Managing change – the art of balancing. *Harvard Business Review*, November-December, 71 (6), 109–118.

East, Central and Southern Africa College of Nursing (ECSACON) (2003) *Report on Evaluation of the ECSA Leadership and Management Programme*. Arusha: ECSACON and the Commonwealth Regional Health Community Secretariat.

Fitzgerald, L.A. (1994) *Living on the Edge*. The Benchmark.

Haines, J. (1993) *Leading in a Time of Change*. Ottawa: Canadian Nurses Association.

Geiger-DuMond, A.H. and Boyle, S.K. (1995) Mentoring: a practitioner's guide in training and development. *Training and Development*, 49 (3), 51.

Greenleaf, R. (1977) *Servant Leader* (1991, 2002), the Robert K. Greenleaf Center for Servant Leadership. NJ: Paulist Press.

Grossman, S.C. and Valiga, T.M. (2000) *The New Leadership Challenge: Creating the Future of Nursing.* Philadelphia: F.A. Davis Company.

Hesselbein, F. (2004) Leadership imperatives in an age of change and discontinuity. Paper presented at the New Zealand Institute of Management Conference, October.

ICN Brochure. *Leadership For Change: An Action-Learning Programme to Develop Nurses as Effective Leaders and Managers in a Constantly Changing Health Environment.* Geneva: ICN.

ICN (1996–2005) Documents for the Leadership for Change program, unpublished.

ICN (2002) (developed by James Buchan). *Impact and Sustainability of the Leadership For Change Project 1996–2000.* Geneva: ICN.

ICN (2004) (developed by Sally Shaw). *Globalisation and Health System Reform: Implications and Strategies for Nursing.* Geneva: ICN.

ICN (2005) *Guidelines on Shaping Effective Health Policy.* Geneva: ICN.

ICN (2005) *Health Policy Package.* Geneva: ICN.

Kanter, R.M. (2005) Interview in *Leader to Leader*, Winter.

Kotter, J.P. (1995) Leading change: why transformation efforts fail. *Harvard Business Review*, March–April.

Kouzes, J.M. and Posner, B.Z. (1995) *The Leadership Challenge.* San Francisco: Jossey-Bass.

Kouzes, J.M. and Posner, B.Z. (1998) *The Leadership Challenge: How to Get Extraordinary Things Done in Organisations*, 2nd ed. San Francisco: Jossey-Bass.

Krueger-Wilson, C. and Porter-O'Grady, T. (1999) Are your management skills obsolete? In: *Leading the Revolution in Health Care: Advancing Systems, Igniting Performance.* Gaithersburg, MD: Aspen Publishers.

Leong, M. *et al.* (2001) *Guidance Through Mentoring.* Booklet prepared by an SNA/ICN LFC™ Project Group. Singapore: Singapore Nurses Association.

Lister, G. (2000) *Global Health and Development: The Impact of Globalization on the Health of Poor People.* UK: The College of Health.

Maina, P.W., Epaalat, D., Munroe, L., Omulogoli, G., Wambua, J., Wanyonyi, J. and Karani, A. (2004). Problems encountered by middle level nurse managers in ensuring quality nursing care in Kenyatta National Hospital. *Kenya Nursing Journal*, 32 (2), 32–36.

Norton, A. and Smythe, L. (2005) *Not Just Another Book About Leadership.* Pre-publication draft.

Nursing in the Caribbean, a Story of Leadership (2002) Publication prepared by Wendy Kitson-Piggott, ICN Regional Project Leader for the Caribbean team. ICN LFC™ publication.

OECD (1994) The Reform of Health Care Systems. *Health Policy Studies.*

Posner, B.Z. and Kouzes, J.M. (1996) Ten lessons for leaders and leadership developers. *Journal of Leadership Studies*, 3 (3), 3.

Rosenbach W.E. and Taylor R.L. (Eds.) (1998) *Contemporary Issues in Leadership*, 4th ed. Colorado: Westview Press.

UNCTAD/UNDP (1999) *Partnership on Globalization, Liberalization and Sustainable Development.*

United Nations (1999) *Globalisation With a Human Face. Overview in Human Development Report.*

University of Nebraska Cooperative Extension (2001) Mentoring. Available at: http://extension.uni.edu/mentoringhome.htm (21 August).

WHO (1993) Health Sector Reform. Report on a Consultation 9–10 December, and (1994) Report on the Second Consultation 28–29 April.

WHO (1993) *Implementation of the Global Strategy for Health Reform by the Year 2000: Second Evaluation.* Geneva: WHO.

Zimmerman, B., Lindberg, C. and Plsek, P. (2001) *Edgeware: Insights from Complexity Science for Health Care Leaders.* Texas: VHA, Inc.

Index